Orthopedic Emergencies:
A Radiographic Atlas

Orthopedic Emergencies: A Radiographic Atlas

Scott V. Haig, MD

Assistant Clinical
Professor of Orthopedic Surgery,
Columbia University,
College of Physicians and Surgeons,
New York, New York
Attending Orthopedic Surgeon
Lawrence Hospital
Bronxville, NY

Carlos R. Flores, MD

Director, Department of Emergency Medicine
Lawrence Hospital
Bronxville, New York

The McGraw-Hill Companies
MEDICAL PUBLISHING DIVISION

New York   Chicago   San Francisco   Lisbon   London   Madrid   Mexico City
Milan   New Delhi   San Juan   Seoul   Singapore   Sydney   Toronto

Orthopedic Emergencies: A Radiographic Atlas

234567890 KGP/KGP 098765

ISBN 0-07-138068-X

This book was set in 10/12, Palatino by Techbooks.
The editors were Andrea Seils, Michelle Watt, and Regina Y. Brown.
The production supervisor was Richard Ruzycka.
Text Design and Layout by Marsha Cohen/Parallelogram Graphics
The index was prepared by Herr's Indexing Service.
KGP was the printer and binder.

This book is printed on acid-free paper.

Library of Congress Cataloging-in-Publication Data

Orthopedic emergencies : a radiographic atlas/edited by Scott V. Haig, Carlos R. Flores.
    p. ; cm.
  Includes index.
  ISBN 0-07-138068-X
    1. Orthopedic emergencies—Atlases. I. Haig, Scott Vanderwink.
  [DNLM: 1. Orthopedic Procedures—methods—Atlases. 2. Emergency Medicine—Atlases.
  WE 17 O77 2004]
  RD732.O755 2004
  616.7'025—dc22
                                                                2003070165

See to it that you do not refuse Him who speaks.

Hebrews 12:25

Contents

Photo
Contributors

Joseph Barmakian, MD

Fellow American Academy of Orthopedic Surgeons
Holder Certificate of Added Qualification in Hand Surgery
Westfield, NJ

Harvey Hecht, MD, FACR, DABR

Stamford Hospital
Stamford, CT

Justin Greisberg, MD

Assistant Professor
Department of Orthopedic Surgery
Columbia University
College of Physicians & Surgeons
New York, NY

Walter Pedowitz, MD

Clinical Professor of Orthopedic Surgery
Department of Orthopedic Surgery
Columbia University
New York, NY

Peter Foley Rizzo, MD

Department of Orthopedic Surgery
Lawrence Hospital,
Bronxville, NY

Robert Strauch, MD

Assistant Professor of Clinical Orthopedic Surgery
Columbia University
New York Presbyterian Hospital
New York, NY

Kristan Zimmerman, MD, DABR

Stamford Hospital
Stamford, CT

Preface

Physicians in emergency departments treat a huge volume of orthopedic injury each year. This book is written to help them in this endeavor. Every effort has been made to make it an entertaining, informative, and attractive volume that is easy to read from cover to cover. Nevertheless, it is our hope that it will found more often at the counter in front of the view box rather than on your favorite chair. This is not an in-depth treatise on fractures; it is guide to help you spot them, treat them, and dispose them properly and quickly.

Limited access to radiologists and orthopedists in smaller hospitals and urgent care centers or during late hours often leaves the emergency practitioner alone with his or her patient, a nonspecific examination (it's tender, swollen, and won't move), and a few plain films. Decision making in such circumstances can be difficult—there are many bone and joint injuries whose radiographic signs are quite subtle. Are the films you have acceptable? Is that bone the trapezoid or the triquetrum? What should you be looking for? What does the normal look like? What are the most common fracture patterns? And then, what should you do about it?

The diagnostic questions need to be answered first. So open the atlas. It is arranged anatomically; the beginning of the appropriate section shows the normal x-rays for that body part with the bones and key joint structures labeled. The criteria for adequacy of the films are here—some structures must be seen despite the unpleasantness of repeating a film.

Next is a list of the problems you can find here, from most common to least, with the radiographic or physical examination clue to expect with them. It's important to know what is common. An awareness of frequency is a large part of the "clinical sense" that we respect in great doctors. That the difficult diagnosis is most often an uncommon presentation of a common problem (think about it) needs to be kept fresh in the mind of everyone who spends their time figuring out what's wrong with sick people.

When you then turn the page, you will be looking at radiographs of the specific fractures. One might look a lot like the case you have up. These cases were picked because the fractures/dislocations were easy to see. The radiographs might not, on the other hand, look anything like your case—in fact, they probably won't. Remember that most orthopedic radiographs made in emergency departments are normal. Even when there is a fracture, it is most frequently nondisplaced and therefore harder to see. You nevertheless should compare your film with the fracture films presented. Seeing our obvious fractures will make your eye more receptive to a more subtle pattern that could be hiding from you in the bluish glare of the view box at four in the morning. If you already have found the fracture on your patient's film, you can then move on to naming it and treating it. But do one more diagnostic check first.

If you do find a fracture on the plain file, the best tool with which to confirm the diagnosis is the index finger of your dominant hand. Tenderness, or specifically, locally maximal tenderness, right on the putative fracture site is a very reliable sign. There are, in fact, a number of fractures for which tenderness is the primary diagnostic criterion—more important than the x-ray. A scaphoid, for example, that is distinctly and reproducibly tender is considered a fractured scaphoid and must be treated as one. This is true of the head of the radius and nearly every growth plate in a child—the tender physis is considered a fracture (termed a *Salter fracture*) even if the x-ray is normal. Therefore, gently press the fracture site with your fingertip. If it is the most tender spot in the area, your x-ray diagnosis is fairly secure. If it is not and there are no reasons for insensitivity to pain, you need to go back to the plain film, considering that what you thought was a fracture probably isn't.

While tenderness is often a big help, it is not of much use in some common emergency situations. Screaming children or unconscious, unresponsive, psychotic, or intubated polytrauma patients make it difficult to find discreet local tenderness. Palpation for tenderness is also of little use in the emergency room classic, the painful hip with a negative x-ray. Calling a negative plain film in a patient with a lot of hip pain is a frequent source of much anxiety to patient, family, and staff . This is so because a patient with any hip fracture needs admission, whereas a patient with acute lumbar radiculopathy, a nondisplaced pelvic fracture, a groin pull, or an arthritic joint usually does not. The hip is one of the few orthopedic areas in which magnetic resonance imaging (MRI) can be essential in the emergency workup. Hip MRIs therefore are included among the fracture photographs, although it is appreciated that many emergency departments have limited access to an MRI unit.

When you have found the fracture pattern most closely fitting your patient, the treatment bullets that go with the photographs will remind you of the essentials of emergency treatment for this particular injury. Some of them are additional diagnostic concerns. Remember that a long bone fracture needs imaging from the joint above to the joint below. An ulnar fracture—any forearm fracture really—requires you to palpate and range the elbow looking for radial head dislocation, a calcaneal fracture needs spine films, and so on. You will be reminded of these each time you open to the fracture photographs. Fractures associated with severe trauma will have laboratory reminders, e.g., complete blood count (CBC), urinalysis (UA), and blood gas determinations for pelvic fractures and comminuted tibia and femur fractures and a chest film and electrocardiogram (ECG) for scapular fractures.

The actual treatments described in these sections are the basics: what needs to be done in the emergency room by the emergency physician. Often, this is fairly bland advice—ice, elevation, a splint or sling, ibuprofen, and see the orthopedist within a certain time frame. In other situations, the treatment may be more exciting— you may need to perform an emergency reduction.

Emergency physicians can and do become adept at reducing fractures and dislocations. Some choose not to. Although personal, financial, and possibly medicolegal factors may suggest waiting for the orthopedist to come in to do the reduction, there will be times in every emergency physician's career when doing the reduction is a must. There are situations in which skin, nerve, or vascular damage becomes worse every minute the deformity persists. There are times when you just can't get the orthopedist. Far more often, though, the emergency physician's decision to do the reduction is simply a matter of humane concern for his or her patient who is in pain that can be relieved only by putting his or her bones back closer to where they belong. It is also generally true that reductions are easier and better when they are done sooner. Of course, you always should keep your orthopedist in the loop.

Most will be more than happy to have you do a reduction—but be sure to make the phone call first. "Would you like me to try?" can prevent a world of hurt.

There is no magic to the reductive maneuvers illustrated in this atlas. You will, however, find them easier when you've actually seen them done. So watch the orthopedist or more experienced emergency room physicians reduce the wrists, ankles, shoulders, and elbows, and ideally, when there is an opportunity, ask the orthopedist to help as you do some. Bear in mind that most of these techniques are taught to beginning orthopedic residents by only slightly more advanced orthopedic residents. Put a few splints on yourself or your coworkers if you've never worked with plaster or fiberglass. While our photographs cannot teach you the feel of a dislocated shoulder clunking in or how tightly to wrap a plaster dressing (looser is better), these are not difficult skills to acquire.

It is presumed that follow-up for an orthopedic problem will be with an orthopedist. The responsible emergency physician needs some control over when this will take place. Communicate with the orthopedist if there is any question as to when or if the patient can be seen; simply giving the patient a phone number invites many chances for error. Remember, the orthopedist on call is burdened to see the patient at your order. If the patient's health plan dictates a visit with the gate-keeping generalist before granting an orthopedic visit, schedule the visit for *tomorrow,* and make sure that the patient knows (and you've documented) that your recommendation is an orthopedic appointment within so many days.

The treatment section for each injury covered in this atlas ends with a disposition comment. Some will be obvious; the patient with an open fracture goes right to the operating room, and the patient with a hip fracture gets admitted to the floor. For others, the proper disposition varies; an overweight older woman who lives alone who presents with an ankle or proximal humerus fracture usually needs admission, whereas a more athletic and capable patient can go home and have further care arranged from there. Those who do go home need clear instructions (*this* takes time!), which include follow-up. Disposition to home therefore includes a time range during which the patient has to see the orthopedist. Again, do not get bogged down with your patient citing a list of health maintenance organization (HMO) stipulations. Insist that the patient get to an orthopedic surgeon within the time you order—this is a medical, not a financial, issue. The patient may choose to go to some other "in plan" surgeon; the appointment in this case is the patient's own responsibility. Nevertheless, it must be within the time frame that you set.

An emergency room physician should address (at least mentally) two issues before sending any orthopedic patient home. First, can the patient perform the activities of daily living (ADLs)? Remember, beside eating, dressing, and toileting, this includes the ability to take care of the injury and such things as being able to elevate, ambulate without bearing weight, and show up for outpatient appointments. Second, would it be best to operate on the patient the next day? If this is the case, even though it is possible to send the patient home, then to the office, then to admitting, then to the floor, and then to the operating room, it is probably still kindest (if not the least expensive) simply to admit the patient through the emergency room for surgery the next day. Good communication with the orthopedist who is to follow the patient is essential here. It is disconcerting to find unknown preoperative patients on one's service during morning rounds.

When a fracture is open (or *compound*), a higher level of urgency attends its treatment. Bone and joint infections are among the hardest to eradicate, and every hour that a fracture stays contaminated increases the risk of infection. The section on open fracture management thus is presented as a quick checklist for you to refer to in addition to the specific fracture section. It is a general section; cultures, antibiotics, immobilization, and initial disinfectants are pretty much the same regardless of a compound fracture's location. The emergency room physician's initial handling of open fractures clearly does make a major difference in their outcomes. This notwithstanding, the call for the ortho-

pedist to come in *now* is also among your first moves with any open fracture. A decision to "wash it out in the emergency room" is a dangerous one and does not belong to the emergency room staff. The great majority of patients with open fractures go immediately to the operating room for irrigation and sharp debridement—this is the orthopedist's job.

Fracture classifications and diagnosis/treatment algorithms are trendy, but they can be great wastes of time. Excellent diagnostic and therapeutic work is done by thousands of physicians with no reference to either of these modern academic preoccupations. Nevertheless, you will be forced to communicate with an orthopedist (probably a resident) at some point who finds it impossible to discuss an orthopedic problem without using a person's name with a number and letter after it. Because of this unfortunate fact, we have, reluctantly, summarized the most important classifications in the appropriate fracture sections. Classifications aren't useless, but their emergency ramifications are limited—so don't worry about learning them. We also give the common eponyms (Jones', Pott's, Smith's, and so on) for those times when you have to call on orthopedists who are really old.

So this is how to use this book: Flip open to the part that hurts, identify the anatomy, find the fracture, and treat it. Fracture cases are satisfying, and you can get better at them with each one you do. Fracture patients usually are grateful for the treatment. We join them in thanking you for the work you do.

*I am grateful to so many who have helped me
during three years spent on this project.*

First the ladies:

Sara Grace Elizabeth – organizational exemplar of perfection
Cecilia Jane Shelmerdine – photographic and computer expert
Stephanie King – ministrations and morale
Johanna Ruzzier, MD – primal fire of science
Helene Gauthier – conscience and protectrix. "You save the World, I'll bill it."
Barbara Arditi – loyal and persistant friend
Melissa Weintraub, MD – At least 7/8th's orthopod
Andrea Seils – steady editorial hand and kind, encouraging voice

And the gentlemen:

Thomas Henry Spencer – focus and enthusiasm
John Samuel Mckenzie – balance, fairness, and computer skills
Thomas L. King – Kindness, generosity, and reason
Armen Charles Haig, MD – The Great One
Carlos Flores, MD – where it all began
Erv Hansen, MD – guiding light

And Charley, Jack, Mike, Greg, Sam, Minas, Tom, Vicky, Esther, and Victoria
who set the whole thing up.

Orthopedic Emergencies: A Radiographic Atlas

1

Toes

ANATOMY (FIG. 1-1)

- Difficult to see on posteroanterior (PA) film, especially if toes are curled. Ask for specific toe films.

- Proximal, middle, and distal phalanges. Hallux = great toe. It has no middle phalanx.
- Base of proximal phalanx is quite proximal to the web space; i.e., the crotch of the web comes down almost to the middle of the proximal phalanx.

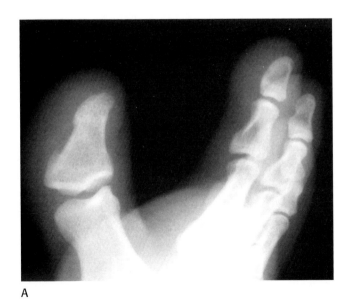

A

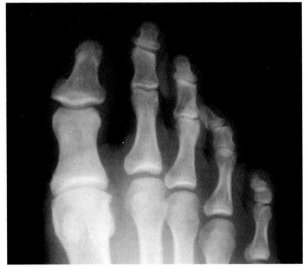

B

FIGURE 1-1

Normal toes. *A.* Posteroanterior (PA) view. *B.* Lateral view.

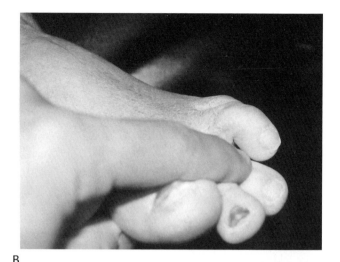

B

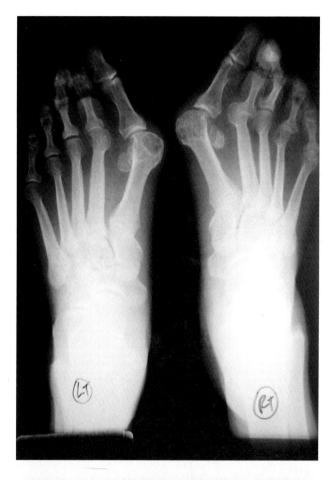

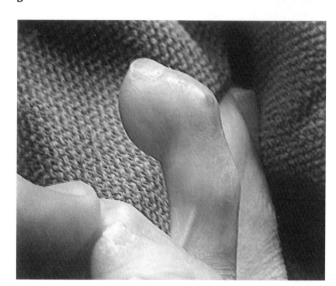

C

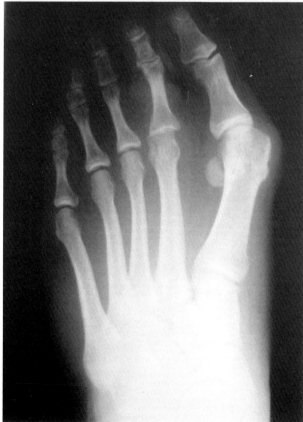

A

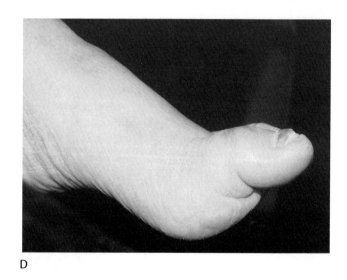

D

FIGURE 1-2

A. Hallux valgus. *B.* Hammer toes. *C.* Mallet toes. *D.* Claw toes.

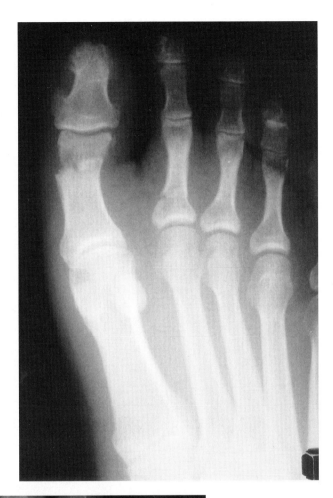

VARIANTS
- Hallux valgus (Fig. 1-2*A*)
- Hammer toes (Fig. 1-2*B*)
- Mallet toes (Fig. 1-2*C*)
- Claw toes (Fig. 1-2*D*)

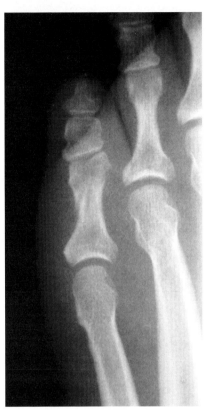

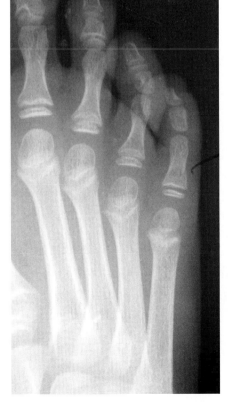

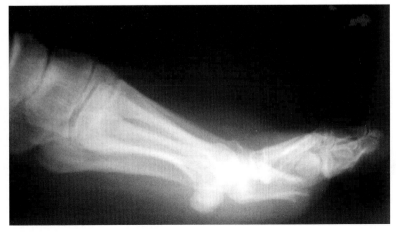

FIGURE 1-3

Fracture, proximal phalanx.

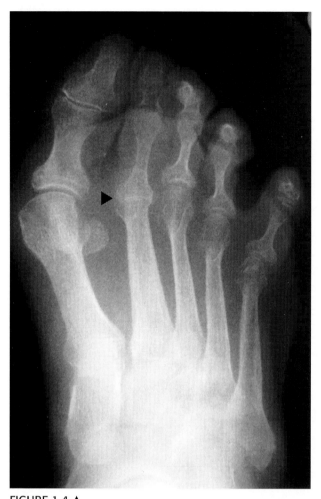

FIGURE 1-4 ▲

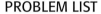

MP dislocation at second metatarsophalangeal joint.

PROBLEM LIST

- Proximal phalanx fracture (stubbing injury) (Fig. 1-3).
- Dislocations of metatarsophalangeal (MP) joint. Do not reduce if chronically dislocated. Claw toes frequently include an MP dislocation (Fig. 1-4).
- Vascular compromise/infection—especially common in diabetics. Call vascular/general surgery.
- Gout. Hallux common, also second toe. Check for history of gout; check urate level. Treat with anti-inflammatory drug and elevation. Medical follow-up. Let the regular physician give the colchicine and allopurinol.
- Middle and distal phalangeal fractures (Fig. 1-5A, B).
- Crush injuries of toes. Often open fractures.
- Subungual hematoma. Can be painful. Drill or burn a 1- to 2-mm hole in the nail plate to relieve pressure, but only if there is intense, throbbing pain. This is a well-known treatment—not often needed.

FIGURE 1-5 ▶

Phalangeal fractures. A. Middle. B. Distal.

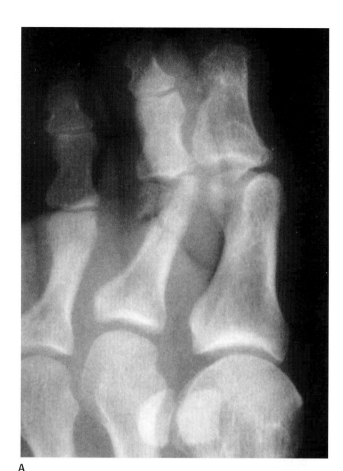

A

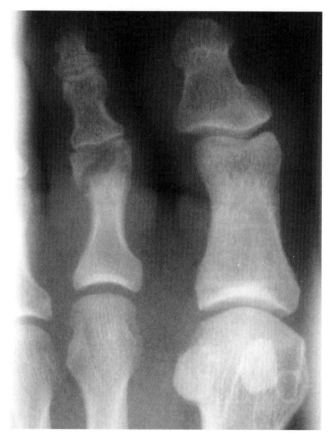

B

TESTS

- Glucose for diabetic/vascular
- Complete blood count (CBC), erythrocyte sedimentation rate (ESR), culture if infection
- Urate if gout is suspected
- Postreduction film
- Neurologic examination of other foot

TREATMENT: DISPLACED FRACTURE

- Straighten it out. Pull and straighten; exaggerate correction. One quick move after thorough icing to numb the toe. A postreduction film is optional.
- Tape if it tends to re-deform. Use plenty of cotton wadding. Keep toe tip visible in any dressing or taping to check circulation.

- Hard, open shoe.
- Crutches.
- Bear weight on heel.
- Tylenol with codeine (these hurt).
- Elevation very important.

DISPOSITION

Discharge home with a 3- to 5-day orthopedic follow-up.

FRACTURE FILMS

- Hallux fracture
- Lesser toe with displacement
- Dislocations

C H A P T E R

2

Metatarsals

NORMAL RADIOGRAPHS

- Posteroanterior (PA) view (Fig. 2-1*A*)
- Lateral view (Fig. 2-1*B*)
- Oblique view (Fig. 2-1*C*)

The bases of the metatarsals are difficult to see. Be suspicious of fractures if there is tenderness here. Get-

ting oblique films at different angles can demonstrate hard-to-see fractures, although treatment does not change. Accessory ossicles have corticated margins and are rounded—the accessory navicular (Fig. 2-1*D*) may be tender after twisting trauma. It is in the tendon of the tibialis posterior.

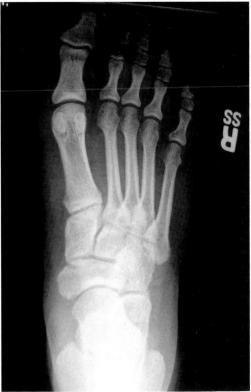
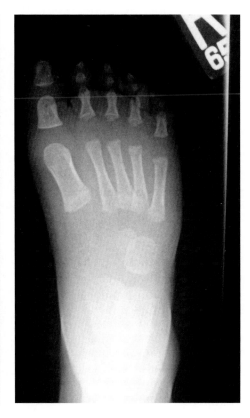

FIGURE 2-1A

Normal foot. *A.* Posteroanterior
(PA) view (*1:* adult; *2:* child).

A

7

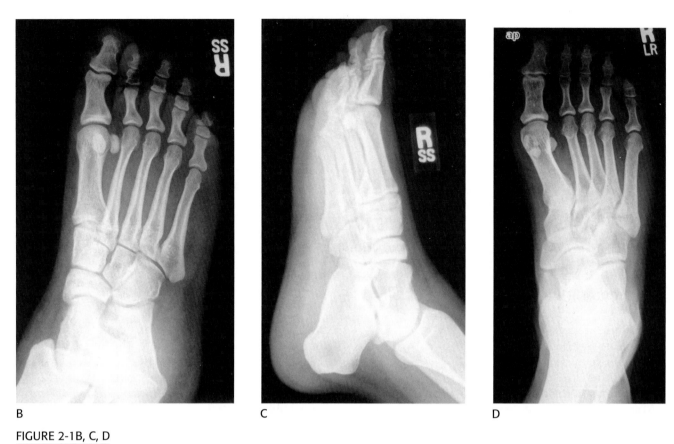

B C D

FIGURE 2-1B, C, D

Normal foot. *B.* Lateral view. *C.* Oblique view. *D.* Posteroanterior view with accessory navicular.

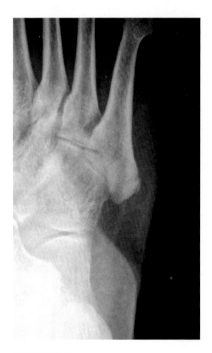
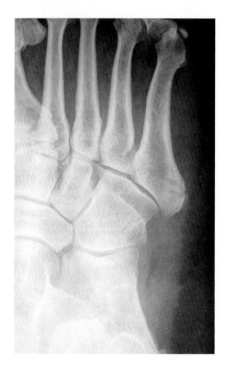
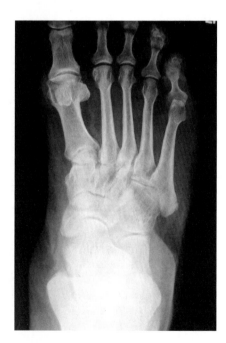

FIGURE 2-2

Fracture of fifth metatarsal base, a "Pseudo-Jones'" fracture.

ANATOMY

The joints at the bases of the metatarsals are called collectively the *Lisfranc joint*.

PROBLEM LIST

- Fifth metatarsal base most common—pseudo-Jones fracture (Fig. 2-2).
- Shaft (Jones fracture). This starts where the cortical wall is discernible; i.e., any diaphyseal component makes it a Jones fracture (Fig. 2-3).
- Metatarsal neck fractures (Fig. 2-4).

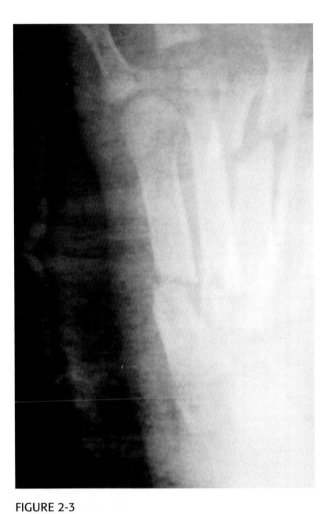

FIGURE 2-3

True Jones fracture.

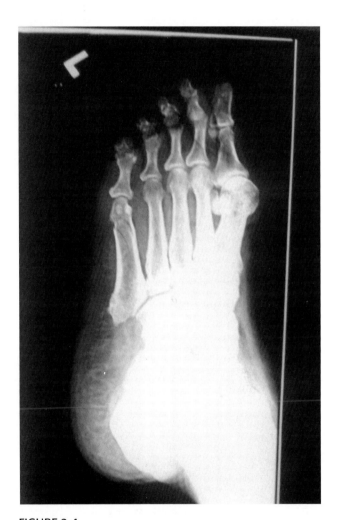

FIGURE 2-4

Metatarsal neck fracture.

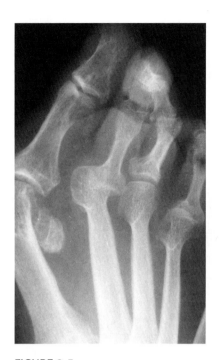
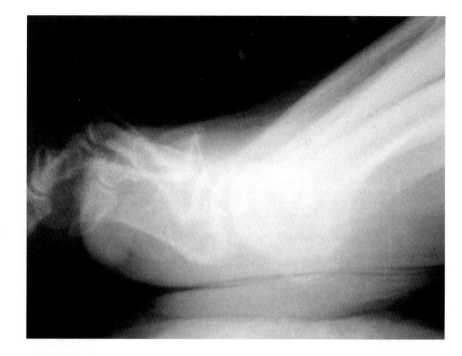

FIGURE 2-5

Metatarsophalangeal (MP) joint dislocation.

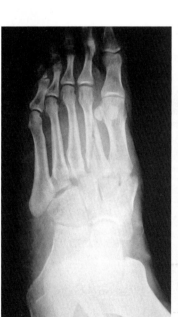
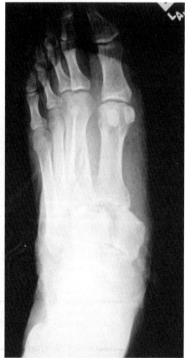
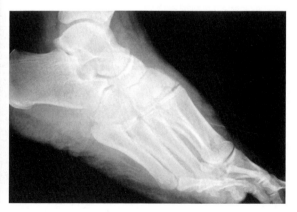

FIGURE 2-6

Tarsometatarsal joint dislocation, a Lisfranc fracture-dislocation.

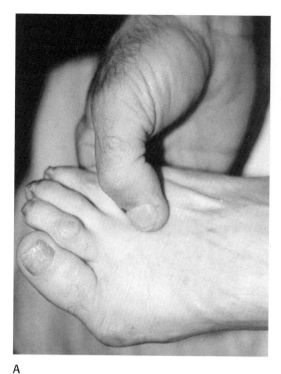

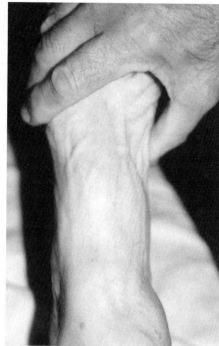

A

B

FIGURE 2-7

A. Morton's pinch. *B.* Morton's squeeze.

- Metatarsophalangeal (MP) dislocations (Fig. 2-5).
- Tarsometatarsal dislocations (Lisfranc dislocations and fracture-dislocations) (Fig. 2-6).
- Intermetatarsal neuroma (Morton's neuroma). Plain film is normal. Pinching the three-quarters (or sometimes the two-thirds) interspace (Fig. 2-7*A*) and squeezing the forefoot (Fig. 2-7*B*) both produce the characteristic pain. Send the patient home with

a hard shoe, ibuprofen, and instructions for elevation and orthopedic follow-up in a week.
- MP joint arthropathy (Fig. 2-8). Same treatment as Morton's neuroma.
- Crush injuries (common) and foot compartment syndromes (unusual but consider when tense swelling is present). Blistering, numbness, and soft tissue loss may indicate admission for strict elevation. Call orthopedics.

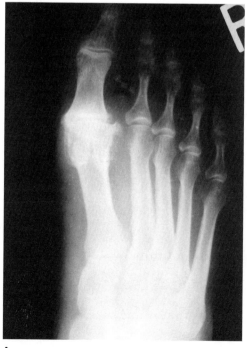

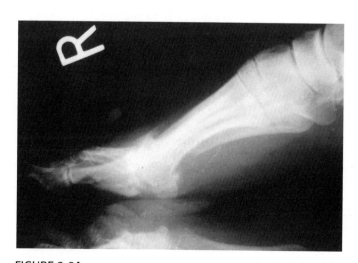

FIGURE 2-8A

A. MP joint arthritis.

A

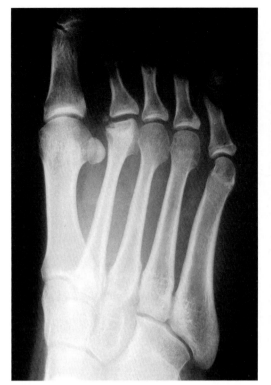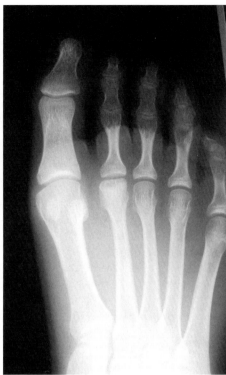

B

FIGURE 2-8B

B. Freiberg's infraction.

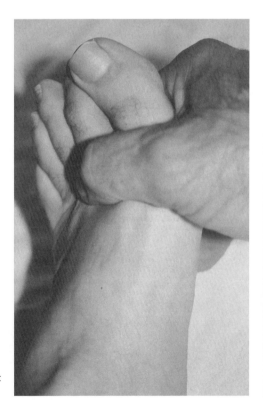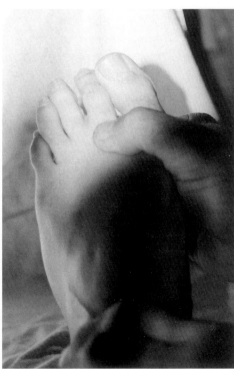

FIGURE 2-9

Reduction of acute MP joint dislocation.

TESTS

- Just make sure that you have sufficient plain-film x-rays. The bases of the metatarsals are often obscured in standard views.
- Do a complete blood count (CBC), erythrocyte sedimentation rate (ESR), and uric acid determination if you are thinking of infection or gout.

TREATMENT

Fractures

- Cast padding and an Ace bandage (a Jones dressing), a hard shoe, and crutches for all.
- A true fifth metatarsal shaft fracture should be nonweightbearing due to high rate of nonunion. These will be casted or internally fixed in many cases.
- Otherwise, weightbearing as tolerated between crutches.
- Elevate; use lots of ice.

MP Joint Dislocations

- Reduce by pushing proximal phalanx with your thumbs off the end of the metatarsal and then down (Fig. 2-9). Do not pull on toe. Must be reduced to be sent home. If you can't get it reduced, call in the orthopedist.
- Beware of chronic dislocations of MP joint with claw toes. Don't think about reducing these—you can't. Check other toes and other foot for comparison. Orthopedist does not need to come in for these.

Tarsometatarsal Fracture/Dislocation—Lisfranc

Elevate, give pain medicine, watch for compartment syndrome, and call in the orthopedist. Patients usually are admitted; often emergency open reduction.

Forefoot Painful without Fracture, Trauma Uncertain

- Rule out infection. Any puncture is assumed to be infected. Patient usually is admitted to medical-surgical unit for intravenous (IV) antibiotics.
- Nonsteroidal anti-inflammatory drugs (NSAIDs), crutches, elevation, and office follow-up within 2 days.
- Intermetatarsal neuroma (Morton's—see above) common.

DISPOSITION

Metatarsal Fractures, MP Joint Dislocations

- Office follow-up within 10 days for all except shaft of fifth.
- Shaft of fifth (Jones): office visit within 3 to 5 days.

Crush Injuries

Admit if compartment suspicion is high or if soft tissue damage/infection risk warrants IV antibiotics. Otherwise, release home with instructions for elevation and non-weightbearing.

SPECIAL CONSIDERATIONS

- Some patients with fifth metatarsal base fractures tolerate an AirCast and are relieved of pain by it. Most don't because its strap presses the fracture site.
- Midfoot pain after waterskiing or horseback riding accidents can be subtle Lisfranc injuries that do not show up on x-rays. No weightbearing and early follow-up for these.

3

Midfoot and Hindfoot

NORMAL RADIOGRAPHS (FIG. 3-1)

- Midfoot: three cuneiforms (•), cuboid (*), navicular (†)
- Hindfoot: calcaneus and talus (os calcis and astragalus to old-timers) (!)

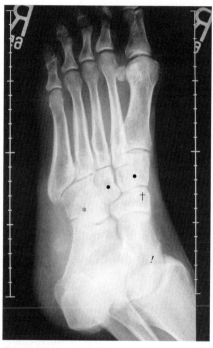

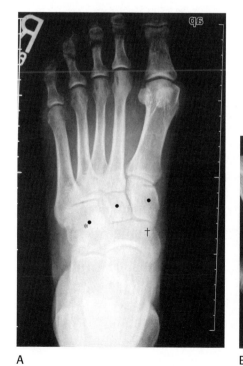

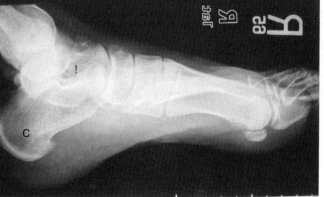

A

B

C

FIGURE 3-1

Normal hindfoot. *A.* Anteroposterior (AP) view. *B.* Lateral view. *C.* Oblique view.

PROBLEM LIST

- Avulsion and impression fractures of talus (Fig. 3-2 *A*), navicular, calcaneus, and cuboid (Fig. 3-2*B*)
- Talar dome, neck, posterior process, body fractures (Fig. 3-3).
- Cuboid nutcracker fracture (Fig. 3-4)
- Calcaneal body fracture (Fig. 3-5)

- Navicular fractures (Fig. 3-6)
- Cuneiform fractures (Fig. 3-7)
- Subtalar dislocations (Fig. 3-8)
- Rupture of spring ligament—films normal, tender plantar midfoot, "top of arch"

FIGURE 3-2

A. Impression fracture of talus. *B.* Avulsion fracture of navicular, calcaneus, cuboid.

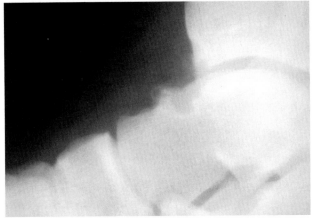

A

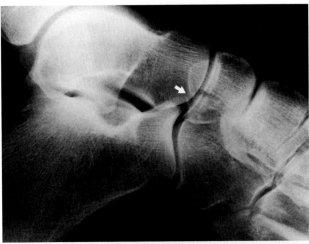

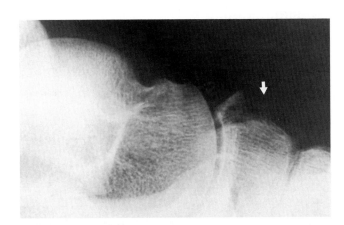

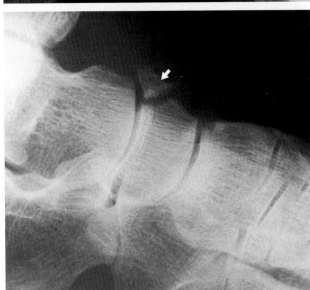

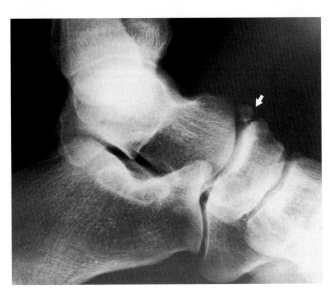

B

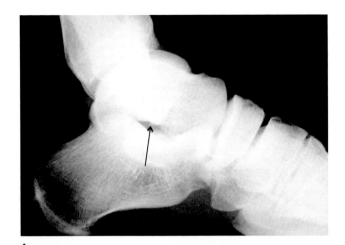

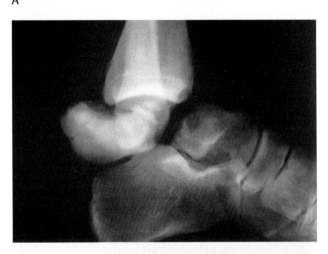

A

FIGURE 3-3

Fractures of the talus. *A.* Dome. *B.* Neck. *C.* Posterior process.

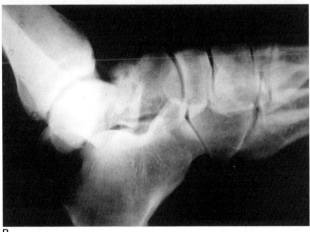

B

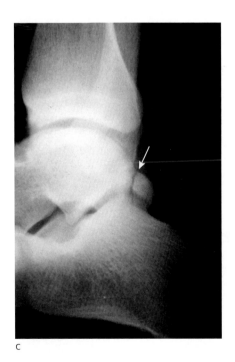

C

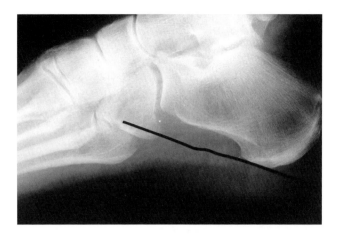

FIGURE 3-4

Fracture of cuboid, nutcracker type.

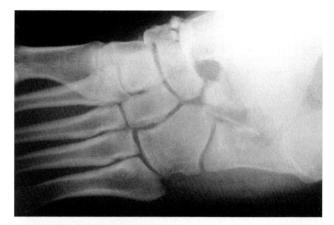

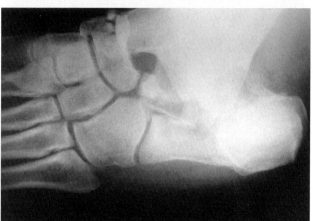

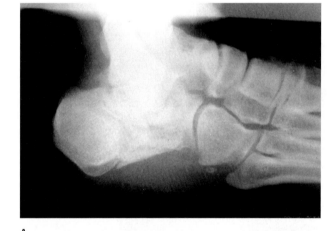

A

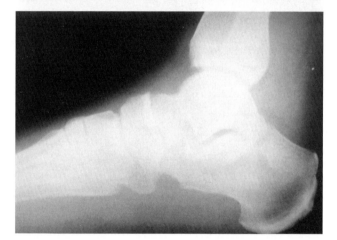

FIGURE 3-6

Fracture of navicular.

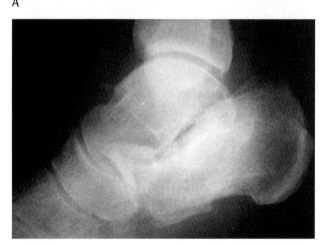

B

FIGURE 3-5

Fracture of calcaneus. *A.* Body. *B.* Anterior process.

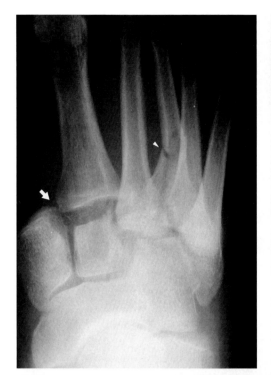
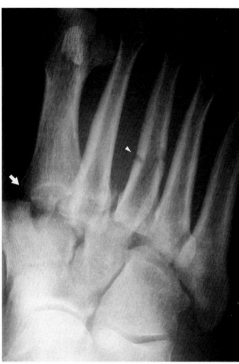

FIGURE 3-7

Fracture of cuneiforms with Lisfranc's dislocation of the tarso-metatarsal joints. Note also third metatarsal shaft fracture.

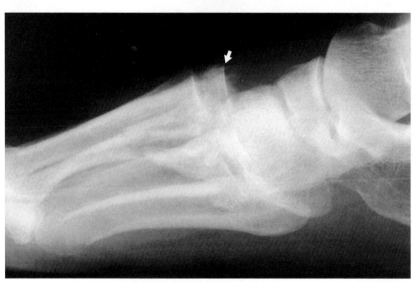

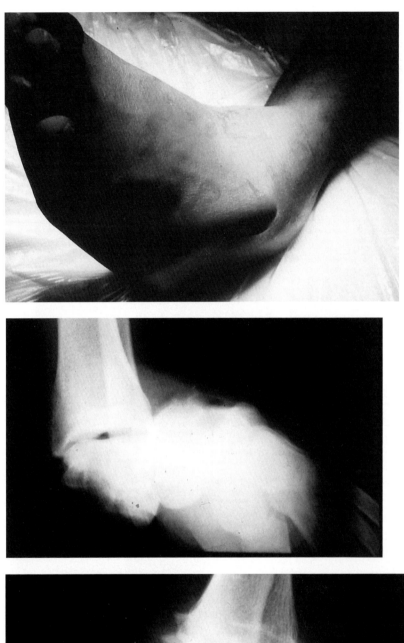

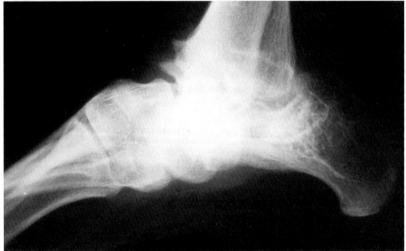

FIGURE 3-8

Subtalar dislocation. Clinical photo, AP and lateral radiographs.

TESTS

Additional plain films are the most frequently useful tests. When the location of maximal tenderness and pain does not seem to suggest a fracture on the initial films, it is often helpful to speak with the x-ray technician about trying oblique or other special views. Many technicians (and their technique books) know how to make hindfoot and midfoot views that bring out otherwise invisible fractures.

Calcaneal fractures are most common in jumpers. Get an AP pelvic film and lumbar spine films, and examine the spine, pelvis, and hips. These are common areas of concomitant fractures.

TREATMENT

- *Avulsion fracture.* A small shell or chunk of bone is ripped away by its attached ligament/tendon. These are *sprains through bone* and are treated with a cotton/Ace dressing, crutches with toe-touch weightbearing, elevation, and ice. A hard shoe is often helpful. Follow-up can be in 10 days because avulsion fractures rarely need casting or internal fixation.
- *Talar neck fracture.* This is most ominous. Any displacement of a talar neck fracture is a true orthopedic emergency. It must be reduced, by the orthopedist, as soon as possible to lessen the likelihood of avascular necrosis. Call the orthopedist in as soon as you make this diagnosis on x-ray. This is not a sufficiently common injury for anyone to have much experience doing the closed reduction. Therefore, call in the orthopedist. He or she will attempt a closed reduction, which generally is accomplished by forceful plantarflexion with a twist into inversion or eversion, depending on the displacement, to bring the head fragment, which moves with the foot, to the neck fragment, which tends to stay with the ankle. These patients usually end up in the operating room for open reduction and screw fixation. Elevate, use ice, and give narcotics in the meantime.
- *Fracture of the talar dome, body, posterior process, and head (the round anterior portion distal to the neck).* This

is less dangerous than a neck fracture. If cleared with the orthopedist, you may send these patients home non-weightbearing with a well-padded posterior mold made from 10 layers of 6-in. plaster wrapped on with more cotton and then an Ace bandage from the toes to the top of the calf with the foot and ankle in a neutral position. Follow-up should be the next day. Elevate, use ice, and make sure that the follow-up is clear. Always tell the orthopedist about these fractures when the patients are in the emergency room. Although infrequent, patients with these fractures sometimes are admitted for surgery.

- *Cuboidal fracture.* This requires cotton/Ace bandage, a hard shoe, non-weightbearing, ice, and elevation. The patient may feel more secure in a posterior mold such as that made for talus fractures above. Follow-up is in up to 7 days.
- *Calcaneal fracture.* First, remember that this is a jumper's fracture with possible head, spine, pelvic, and visceral injury. Second, such fractures all swell tremendously—so no constrictive dressings. Very loose cotton/Ace bandage, non-weightbearing, strict elevation, and ice for 48 hours. These are often very painful, and patients often are admitted, so be sure to inform the orthopedist before sending the patient home.

Making a Well-Padded Posterior Mold Splint (Fig. 3-9)

1. Measure plaster; use a 6-in plaster of Paris roll.
2. Use 10 layers minimum.
3. Use four layers of cotton padding.
4. Wrap on with cotton and then an Ace bandage.

CLASSIFICATION

THE HAWKINS CLASSIFICATION OF TALAR NECK FRACTURES

1. Nondisplaced vertical crack in neck of talus
2. Displaced or comminuted neck of talus
3. Dislocation of body of talus—severe trauma, usually open

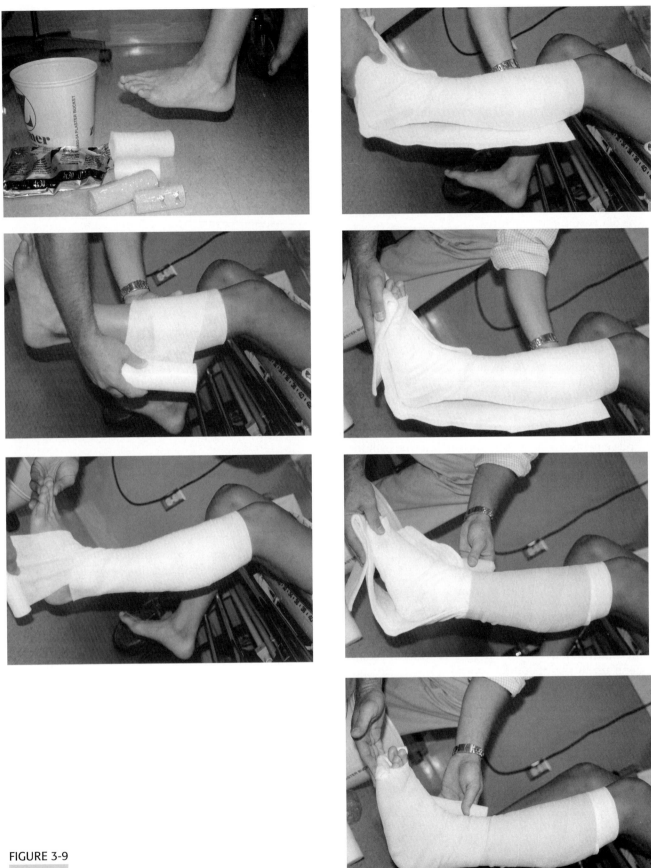

FIGURE 3-9

Making a posterior mold splint.

4

Ankle and Distal Tibia

NORMAL RADIOGRAPHS

Normal radiographs include anteroposterior (AP) (Fig. 4-1A), lateral (Fig. 4-1B), and mortise views (Fig. 4-1C). The mortise view is important because it shows the joint space on both the medial and lateral sides of the talus. You must have this view on every ankle case—fractures and ligament injuries will be missed if you only get AP and lateral views.

ANATOMY

- Tibia (t), fibula (F), talus (τ)
- Medial (m), lateral (L), and posterior malleoli (P). (The posterior malleolus is just the slight downward lipping of the back of the distal tibia, seen on the lateral view; it is not a palpable bump like the medial and lateral malleoli are.)
- Plafond (Pl), talar dome (D)
- Posterior process of talus. (Note that the flexor tendon of the big toe passes through this; when you think this process may be fractured, moving the big toe actively or passively produces pain (Pp) in the hindfoot.)
- Colliculi of lateral malleolus (where the anterior talofibular ligament and the posterior talofibular ligament attach to the fibula). (Small, hard to see avulsion fractures of the colliculi are picked up by noting true bony tenderness of the fibula.)
- Anterior talofibular ligament (ATFL), posterior talofibular ligament (PTFL), calcaneofibular ligament (CFL), deltoid ligament (see 4-11).

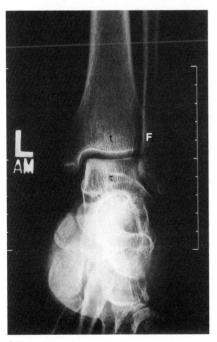
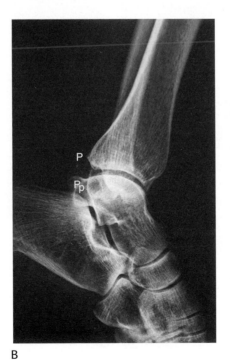
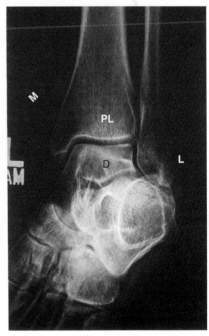

A   B   C

FIGURE 4-1

Normal ankle. *A.* Anteroposterior (AP) view. *B.* Lateral view. *C.* Mortise view.

PROBLEM LIST

Ligament Injuries ("Sprains")

- Lateral ligament—the typical "sprained ankle"
- Radiographs are normal (may see soft tissue swelling)

Disruption of the Tibial-Fibular Interosseous Ligament

Radiographs may show subtle to pronounced widening of the mortise (Fig. 4-2). This means that the medial or lateral joint space is wider than the superior joint space.

- *Syndesmotic rupture.* The syndesmosis is the tough ligamentous connection between the tibia and fibula. Also called the *tibial-fibular interosseous ligament.* Injury to the syndesmosis lets the two bones spread apart, widening the mortise of the ankle. This lets the talus move side to side excessively, predisposing to arthritis.
- Watch out for a high fibular shaft fracture when the mortise is widened. The break in the fibula is often above the top of the film, so palpate the whole length of the fibula, right up to the knee, and get films of any portion that is tender.
- Deltoid (medial) ligament injury.

Rupture of Achilles Tendon

Don't miss this. The plain-film radiograph frequently is normal. Often there is not much pain, and the patient can walk with an externally rotated leg, disguising lack of push-off strength. Remember, the toe

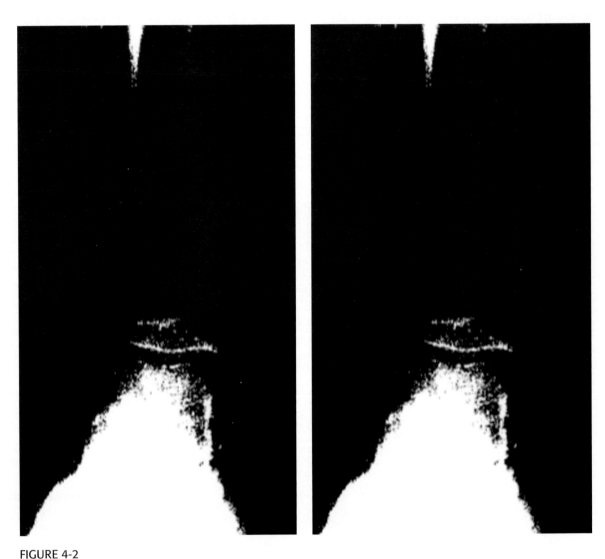

FIGURE 4-2

Widened mortise, no fracture.

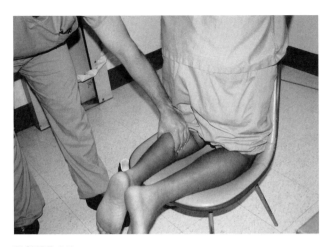

FIGURE 4-3

Thompson's test.

flexors and tibialis posterior can still give some weak plantarflexion despite complete loss of the Achilles tendon. Thompson's test (Fig. 4-3) is quite reliable. Have the patient kneel on a soft chair and relax both legs. Squeeze the uninjured side of the calf and watch how the ankle and foot move. Now squeeze the affected side of the calf. If there is a ruptured Achilles tendon, the motion will be much less. It is also usually possible to palpate the "divot" where the rupture is. Distinguish this from a higher calf tear, which is a musculotendinous junction tear of the medial head (lateral is rare) of the gastrocnemius. These patients have a sudden calf pain but still have fairly normal plantarflexion strength. Their Thompson's test is nearly normal (the ankle moves almost as well as the good side when the calf is squeezed), and there is a tender spot in the medial belly of the calf. Patients with both types of injuries are treated with crutches, weight-bearing as tolerated, and next day orthopedic follow-up. The distal tendon tear is best treated surgically.

Fractures

- Avulsion fractures: tip of the fibula, cuboid avulsion, posterior talar process (Fig. 4-4)
- Lateral malleolus fractures, i.e., fractures of the fibula at the ankle (Fig. 4-5)
- Medial malleolus fractures (Fig. 4-6)
- Bimalleolar fractures (distal fibula and medial malleolus) (Fig. 4-7)
- Trimalleolar fractures (bimalleolar and posterior tibial lip) (Fig. 4-8)
- Pilon fractures (talus smashes upward into distal tibia, breaking the "ceiling" or plafond of the tibia) (Fig. 4-9)

- Triplane or Tilleaux fractures. A vertical fracture of the distal tibial epiphysis is the hallmark of these. This vertical lucency in the tibia just above the ankle joint line can be difficult to see on the AP and even on the mortise views. Suspect these in any child or teen with weight-bearing pain and tenderness of the distal tibia (Fig. 4-10).

TESTS

Be ready to take Doppler pulses in the foot when swelling and injury make loss of distal circulation a concern. If no pulses are detectable, do the reduction and recheck. If there still are no pulses, call in orthopedist stat.

Rapid reduction, even "part of the way back," can save endangered skin and lessen soft tissue ischemia or stretch injury. Make sure to get postreduction films.

Make sure to palpate the entire length of the fibula from knee to ankle looking for tenderness. A fibula fracture produced by a twisting injury of the ankle can be as high as the knee.

The squeeze test is done by squeezing the fibula to the tibia 8 in. or so above the ankle. If this maneuver produces pain in the lateral part of the ankle, there is probably a disruption of the syndesmosis (or a fibula fracture) even if the x-ray is normal.

TREATMENT

Ligament Injuries

These are most common. Patients are almost always tender just anterior to the distal fibula in the "soft spot" (where the acute swelling usually is) (Fig. 4-11). An AirStirrup is great. Use over a smooth sock or smoothly wrapped Ace bandage. Teach the patient how to apply it. Patients should remove it to wash, dry, and let the skin breathe. Crutches, partial weightbearing, ice, elevation, and ibuprofen or Tylenol 3 are appropriate. The patient may wear a loose shoe with an AirStirrup. If you cannot get an AirStirrup, make a Jones dressing with cotton/Ace/cotton/Ace to produce a bulky and stiff "soft cast" from the toes to 8 in. above the ankle. Follow-up should be within 1 week.

Fractures

- *Avulsion fractures* are *ligament injuries through bone.* Treat as under "Ligament Injuries" above.
- Any dislocation needs to be reduced immediately. This is not difficult. Remember to clear this with the orthopedist on call. Anesthetize with 10 ml of 1%

FIGURE 4-4

Avulsion fracture. *A.* Fibula tip. *B.* Cuboid (*). *C.* Posterior talar process.

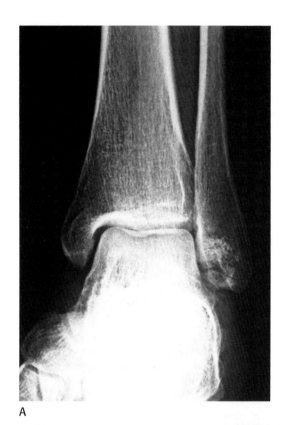

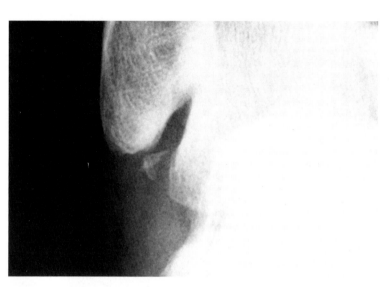

A

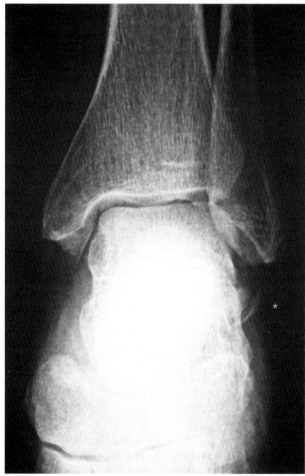

B

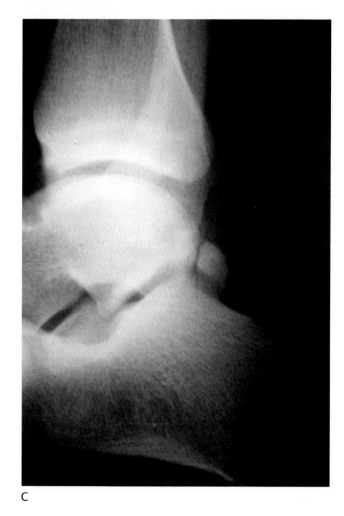

C

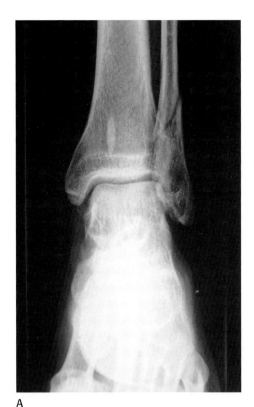

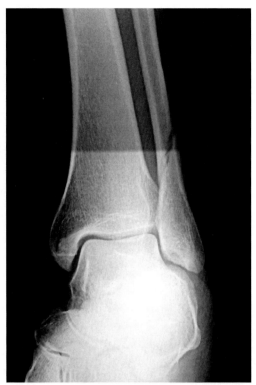

A

FIGURE 4-5

Lateral malleolus fracture. *A.* Mortise view. *B.* Lateral view. *C.* High fibula, Maisonneuve type.

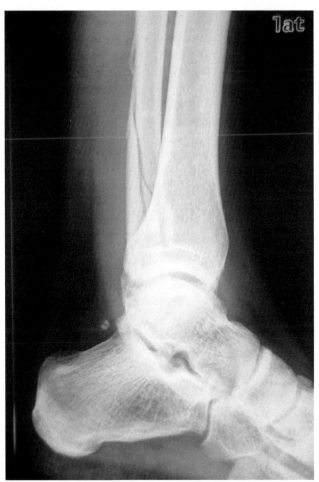

B

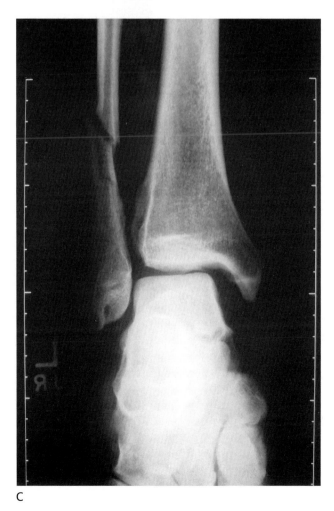

C

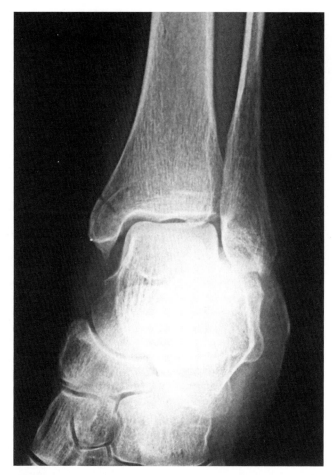

FIGURE 4-6

Medial malleolus fracture. Mortise view.

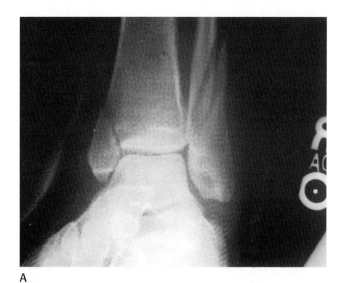

A

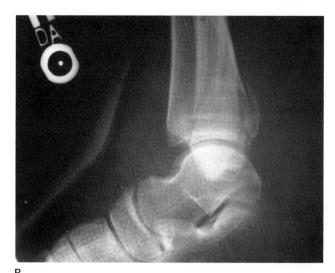

B

FIGURE 4-7

Bimalleolar fracture. *A.* Mortise view. *B.* Lateral view.

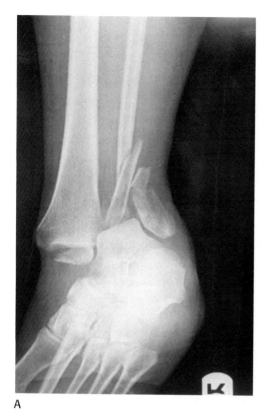

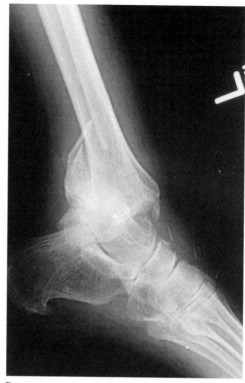

A

B

FIGURE 4-8

Trimalleolar fracture. *A.* Mortise view. *B.* Lateral view.

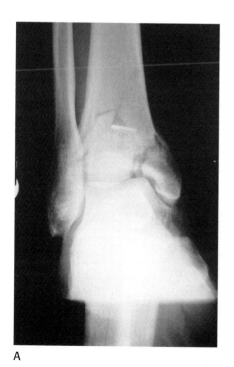

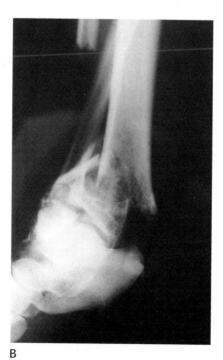

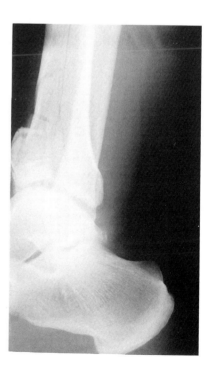

A

B

FIGURE 4-9

Pilon fracture. *A.* Anteroposterior (AP) view. *B.* Lateral view.

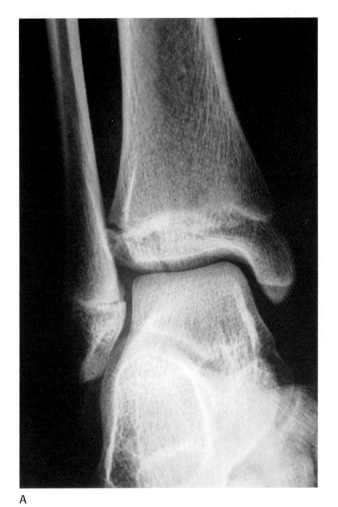

A

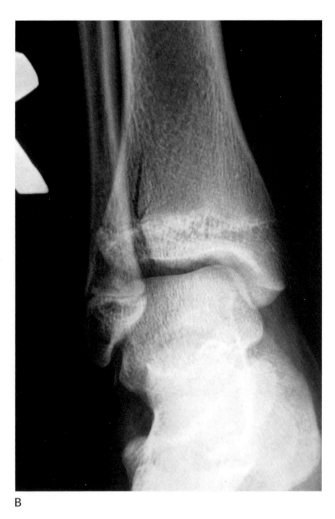

B

FIGURE 4-10

Tilleaux fracture. Mortise view.

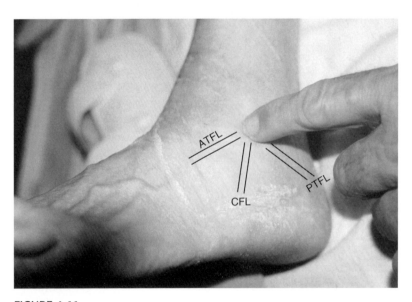

FIGURE 4-11

Anterior talofibular ligament (ATFL) tender spot.

lidocaine (no epinephrine) after prepping the skin with Betadine and then alcohol. Inject into the joint space. Wait 10 min, and then reduce by exaggerating the deformity, applying traction, then putting the talus/foot back into place under the tibia. Splint with a posterior mold of 10 layers of 6-in. plaster padded with five layers of cotton and wrapped on from calf to toes with more cotton and then an Ace bandage (see Fig. 3-9). Not too tight—they all swell.

- *Lateral malleolus fractures* often require open reduction and internal fixation. Contact the orthopedist. He or she may want to admit the patient for next day surgery. When the fracture is not widely displaced (i.e., displacement is less than the width of the fibula), a competent patient can be sent home non-weightbearing in a posterior mold (see above) or AirStirrup with next day follow-up.
- *Bimalleolar fractures.* Orthopedists usually are more comfortable admitting patients with these fractures in order to elevate prior to surgery. Put the patient into a posterior mold after doing a provisional reduction, and send the patient up to the floor with the ankle iced and elevated on three pillows. An athletic patient with less than a centimeter of fracture displacement may go home in a posterior mold, non-weightbearing, with next day follow-up if the orthopedist is agreeable.
- *Medial malleolus only.* An AirStirrup (not too tight on fracture site), toe-touch weight-bearing, ice, analgesics, and follow-up within 48 h are acceptable if the orthopedist does not want to admit the patient for next day surgery.
- *Trimalleolar.* Generally, admit the patient for surgery when swelling permits. Provide extra cotton padding/wrapping on splint, strict elevation, and lots of narcotic.
- *Pilon.* This is a truly miserable fracture to treat. Patients can be 4 months non-weightbearing after a difficult and risky internal fixation procedure. Splint and admit.
- *Triplane and Tilleaux.* These are uncommon but not rare. These are fractures of the distal tibial epiphysis and physis in children and young adults. The epiphysis is the tibial plafond or joint surface. The subtle gap in the plafond is best seen on a mortise or AP view of the ankle (Fig. 4-9*A,B*). A posterior mold splint, non-weightbearing ambulation and 12-h orthopedic or pediatric-orthopedic follow-up

is needed. Many are admitted directly for surgery as growth disturbance is a concern.

Reduction

As described earlier, lidocaine injected into the joint is a good analgesic for reduction. Lifting and holding the foot by the toes (with patient supine) pulls the talus forward and tends to apply an internal rotation force to the talus because of the natural tendency of the hips to rotate externally. These forces tend to reduce most displaced ankle fractures. It is also easy to wrap on the splint or cast while an assistant is holding the toes.

Take one or two tries at reduction, and get a postreduction film. If the talus is not going back under the tibia, there is a good chance that the tibialis posterior tendon has fallen into the joint, the peronei are in spasm, or the deltoid ligament is preventing reduction. This means that the reduction cannot be achieved outside the operating room—so stop trying, splint it where it lies, and call in the orthopedist.

SPECIAL CONCERNS

Ankle fractures and ligament injuries all swell tremendously for a long time. Warn the patient about this repeatedly—explain the importance of elevation and how to loosen dressings if they feel too tight. In patients with peripheral vascular disease, this is compounded. Avoid ice if the foot has stigmata of vascular insufficiency.

CLASSIFICATION

There are many systems, but the one most people remember is Weber's for bimalleolar and trimalleolar fractures.

Weber A: Fibula fracture distal to tibial plafond
Weber B: Fibula fracture at same level as plafond
Weber C: Fibula fracture proximal to plafond

Potts fracture is used by old-timers for bimalleolar fractures. *Maisonneuve fracture* means a very high fibula fracture produced by twisting of the foot—syndesmosis rips up until it "breaks out" at the fracture site.

5

Tibia and Fibula Shaft

NORMAL RADIOGRAPHS (FIG. 5-1)

The tibia is the big bone, and the fibula the small one (although the "tibula" and "fibia" remain favorites on television doctor shows).

PROBLEM LIST

Fracture of the Tibial Shaft with Fibular Fracture (the "Tib-Fib" Fracture)

This is the classic "broken leg." Almost all patients require admission, at least overnight. This injury is seen commonly in multiple trauma, so examine the patient carefully for foot and ankle injuries, as well as pelvic, spine, head, and visceral problems.

A common error is to mistake a nutrient artery of the tibia for a non-displaced fracture. These "nutrient arteries" are oblique radiolucencies that do not produce local tenderness to palpation. If the crack you are looking at is tender call it a fracture and let the orthopedist and radiologist decide if it could be an artery through the cortex.

If there is a break in the skin of the leg that probes down to bone with a sterile cotton applicator (which might as well be a culture swab because you need to culture the wound anyway), you have a true surgical emergency. This patient goes right to the operating

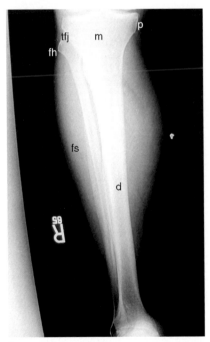
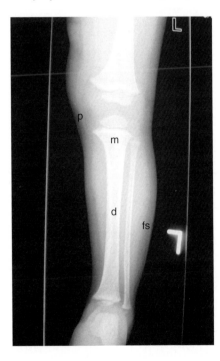
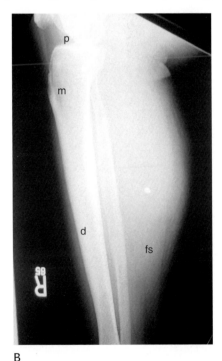

A
B

FIGURE 5-1

Normal tibia. *A.* Anteroposterior (AP) view. *B.* Lateral view. m = metaphysis of tibia; d = diaphysis of tibia; p = plateau of tibia; fs = fibula shaft; fh = fibula head; tfj = tibia-fibula joint.

room for cleansing and must be started on intravenous (IV) antibiotics as soon as cultures have been taken.

Compartment syndromes of the leg are fairly common with tibia fractures. A diagnostic difficulty is that the early clinical signs of pain, tense swelling, and pain with passive motion of the toes all can be produced simply by the fracture. When its really compartment syndrome, the pain and tenseness are truly severe. This is when surgical fasciotomy should be done. Waiting for neurologic and/or vascular loss to do the release is waiting too long.

Measuring compartment pressure, unless you do it all the time, is tricky, even with the special devices made for this. Do not be talked into "ruling out" compartment syndrome with one of these devices when the clinical signs point to it.

Compartment syndrome is a vascular problem. It is treated by vascular surgeons or general surgeons in many community hospitals but by orthopedic surgeons in most teaching hospitals. When the fracture is to undergo surgical stabilization, the orthopedist certainly can do the fasciotomy but may want a "soft tissue person" to take care of the open wound that the fasciotomy leaves. In any case, the potential for time wasting is tremendous. Compartment syndrome is quite serious. If you have any concern that time will be wasted as the services bicker, it is safest to call them both in stat.

The orthopedist needs to come in for every fractured tibia, even completely nondisplaced ones. Some patients can be casted in the emergency room and sent home. Many get admitted for observation of circulatory status overnight. Patients also may request intramedullary rodding, which obviates casting, when they find out how long the cast would stay on (although cast treatment is perfectly legitimate in most cases).

Fractures of the Shaft, Head of Fibula (Fig. 5-2)

This diagnosis can be made only if you are sure there is nothing wrong with the ankle. The story here is of a direct blow to the lateral aspect of the leg. The patient usually can walk on the leg, and tenderness is localized.

The fracture may be visible on one view only. An internal-rotation view of the knee (like the mortise view of the ankle) shows small fractures of the fibular head better than the straight anteroposterior (AP) view. Get this if there is pain and tenderness of the fibular head but no fracture is seen on the AP and lateral views. The fibula is also an inconspicuous bone. Small fibula fractures are easily overlooked when big tibia and femur fractures are nearby (Fig. 5-2C).

Peroneal nerve palsy with a foot drop (this means the inability to dorsiflex the ankle) and numbness on the dorsum of the foot is a common finding with fibula shaft fractures. This is from direct trauma to the

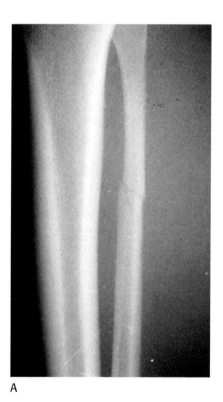

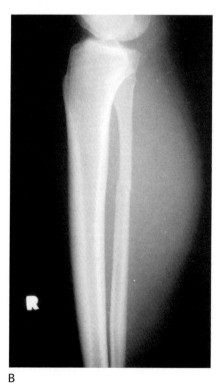

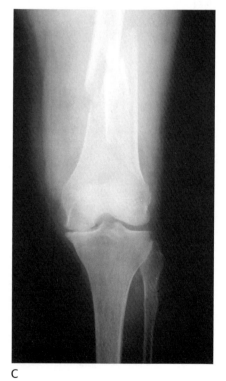

A   B   C

FIGURE 5-2

Fibula shaft fracture. *A.* Anteroposterior (AP) view. *B.* Lateral view. *C.* Surprise with femur shaft.

peroneal nerve, which is palpable as it wraps around the shaft of the fibula 1 to 2 in. below the head of the fibula.

Compartment syndrome is possible with fibular shaft fractures, especially if the patient is on warfarin (Coumadin). This is not common.

TESTS

Measure compartment pressure. As mentioned earlier, this gets academic quickly. At best, it is a confirmatory test. If you don't have one of the little electric devices, a lumbar puncture set works just fine. Just bear in mind that if you are thinking this seriously about a compartment syndrome, the orthopedist on call should be there already.

Take Doppler pulses if you cannot palpate them. Straightening out a very crooked leg can improve poor distal circulation. Remember, having pulses does not mean that you do not have a compartment syndrome brewing. Tenseness, pain in the leg with passive motion

of the toes, worsening or intolerable pain (the pain of ischemia), and later, loss of light touch sensation in the foot are signs of compartment syndrome that you need to look for.

If the bone is sticking out and is grossly contaminated, it needs to be debrided and washed thoroughly before being put back into the leg. This is the surgeon's job. Culture it beforehand.

Tibia fractures are dramatic, dominating the patient's and possibly your own attention. Don't forget the joints above and below, as well as the rest of the trauma workup for head, neck, viscera, and so on.

TREATMENT

Tibial Shaft Fractures (Figs. 5-3, 5-4, and 5-5)

Arrange for admission in most cases. Immobilize and elevate the limb, provide narcotics, and await arrival of the orthopedist. This is generally the routine for closed fractures.

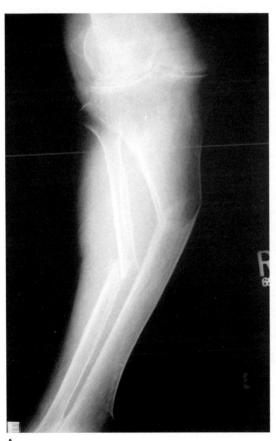 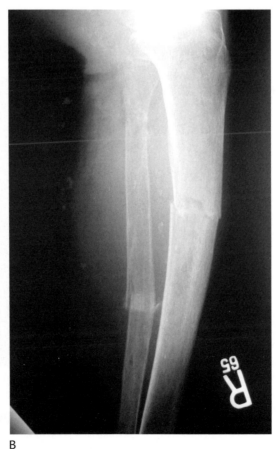

A   B

FIGURE 5-3

Tibia-fibula fracture, low-energy injury in soft bone. *A.* AP view. *B.* Lateral view.

FIGURE 5-4

Tibia-fibula fracture, moderate-energy injury in normal bone. *A.* AP view. *B.* Lateral view.

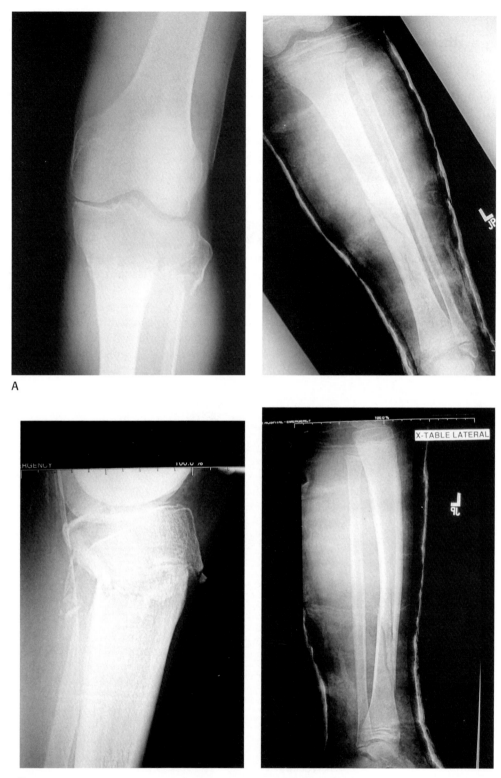

A

B

Open fractures need an IV access, culture of the wound, a Betadine dressing applied to the wound, and *then* an IV antibiotic. Immobilize and elevate the limb, and give pain medicine as the antibiotic is going in. Protocols vary for which drugs to use, but 1 to 2 g cephazolin generally is safe to start with in patients with a small (<2 cm) compounding wound. A large, dirty wound needs two or three antibiotics to achieve anaerobic and gram-negative coverage. Ciprofloxacin (750 mg) in addition to the cephazolin is one safe way of doing this.

Reduction and casting of tibia-fibula fractures are done by the orthopedist unless you are greatly

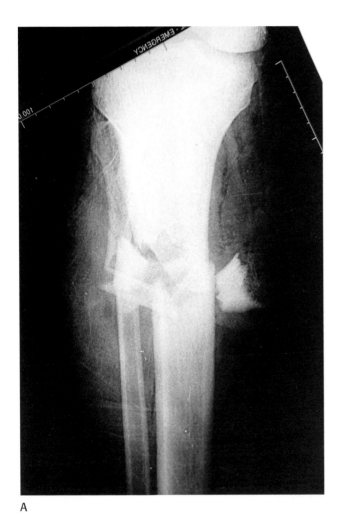

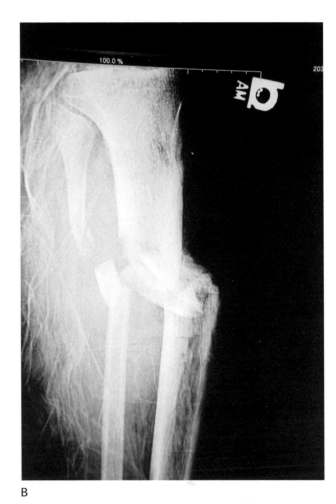

A

B

FIGURE 5-5

Tibia-fibula fracture, high-energy injury in hard bone (compartment syndrome case). *A.* AP view. *B.* Lateral view.

experienced in putting on casts. The splint applied in the emergency department is primarily for comfort and ease in transferring the patient. See Fig. 3-9 for how to apply a posterior mold splint. A knee immobilizer often is adequate. Do not wrap anything tightly around the leg. Do elevate the leg on one or two pillows. Use a lot of ice.

Fibula Shaft or Head Fractures

Patients with this type of fracture can go home with crutches, with Tylenol 3, weightbearing as tolerated, ambulation, and ice. Document peroneal nerve function. Although unnecessary, an Ace bandage wrapped loosely around the fracture site makes the patient feel

that you "did something" for the fracture. Follow-up occurs in 2 to 7 days.

CLASSIFICATION

The open fracture classification of Kyle and Gustilo is used most often to describe open tibia-fibula fractures.

Type 1: Compounding wound of <1 cm in maximum dimension
Type 2: 2- to 10-cm wound
Type 3: >10-cm wound or any really nasty, tissue-destroying, dirty wound

See Chap. 18, "Open Fractures."

6

Knee: Proximal Tibia

NORMAL
RADIOGRAPHS
(FIGS. 6-1 AND 6-2)

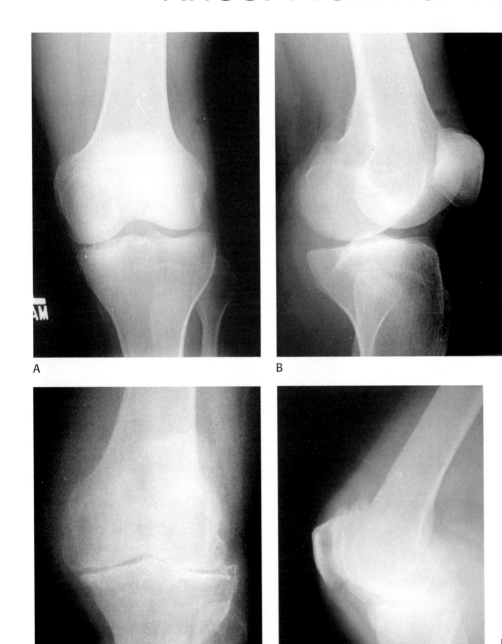

A

B

C

D

FIGURE 6-1

A. Normal knee, anteroposterior (AP) view. *B.* Lateral view. *C.* Arthritic knee, AP view. *D.* Lateral view.

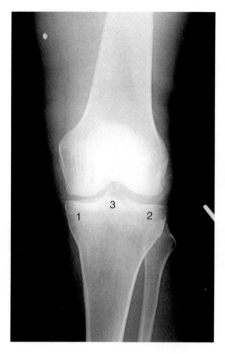
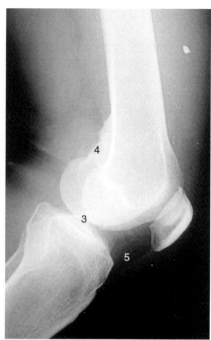

FIGURE 6-2

Normal knee, long view. Medial (1), lateral plateau (2), intercondylar eminence of tibial spine (3), fabella (4), joint lines (5) seen on lateral.

PROBLEM LIST

Medial or Lateral Plateau Fractures

- *Insufficiency type* (Fig. 6-3). A very mild depression of the joint surface is seen. Sometimes this is diagnosed only by specific local tenderness and then a bone scan or magnetic resonance imaging (MRI) showing the fracture (i.e., the plain film fails to show fracture). The knee can be full of blood. Subtle depression or compaction of bone seen on most if film is well centered at the joint line. There is much pain when patient attempts to bear weight—this is the primary diagnostic clue. These are fractures of weak bone. Little or sometimes no trauma is noted in the history.

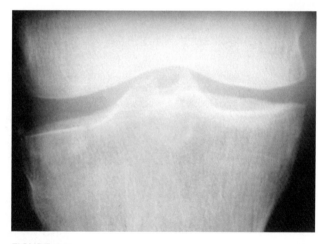

FIGURE 6-3

Fracture of the medial plateau, insufficiency type.

- MRI will show this fracture much more dramatically, and indeed, there are many such fractures that simply do not show up on plain films but are easily seen on MRI. Since no major *emergency* management decision hinges on the presence or absence of this nondisplaced fracture, emergency MRI of the suspected plateau fracture is not an absolute necessity (as it often is in the case of plain-film-negative hip fractures).

- *Depressed type* (Fig. 6-4). There is an obvious dent in plateau made by the femoral condyle. Some deformity of knee is present—varus for the medial plateau, valgus for the lateral. These fractures always have a bloody effusion. There is some risk of compartment syndrome.

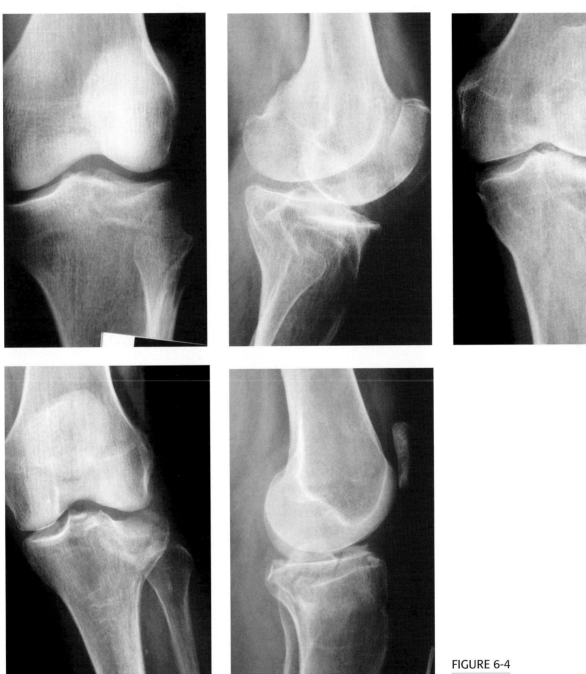

FIGURE 6-4

Fracture of the tibial plateau, depressed type.

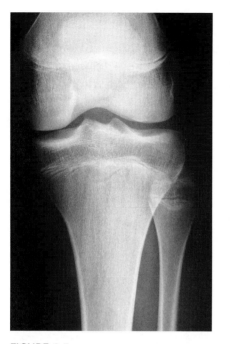
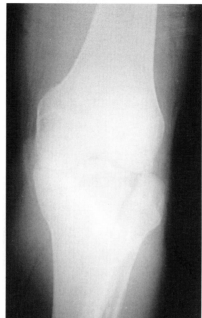
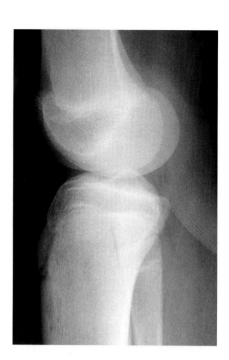

FIGURE 6-5

Fracture of the tibial plateau, split type.

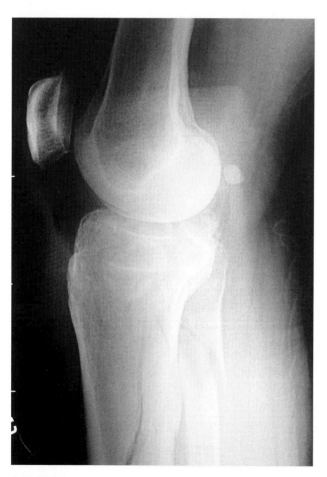
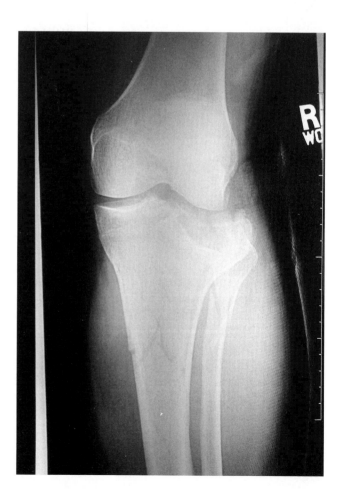

FIGURE 6-6

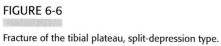

Fracture of the tibial plateau, split-depression type.

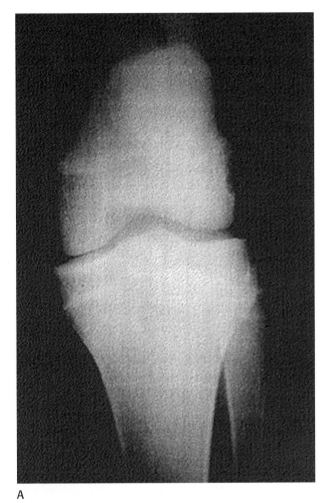

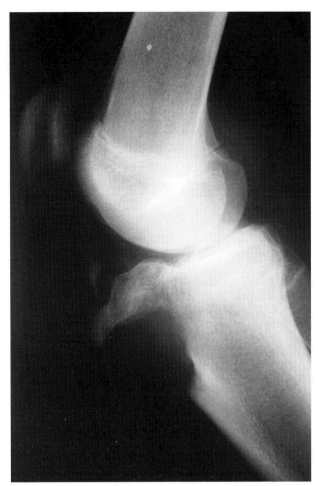

A   B

FIGURE 6-7

A. Tibial tubercle fracture, AP view. *B.* Lateral view.

- *Split type* (Fig. 6-5). A chunk of the upper tibia is cloven away. When such a fracture is nondisplaced, vertical fracture lines extend into the tibial metaphysis. Varus/valgus deformity is a common feature, as well as tight effusion. The knee obviously is very unstable.
- *Split-depression type* (Fig. 6-6). There is a significant chunk off the joint or a vertical fracture line, as well as crushing, denting, or depression of the articular surface.

Tibial Tubercle Fractures (Fig. 6-7)

This is an avulsion caused by the pull of the patellar tendon. The special anatomy of this epiphysis is seen in the lateral view (see Fig. 6-7*B*). Beware of Osgood-Schlatter tibial apophysitis—this is a chronic condition in 10- to 15-year-olds that might get especially painful after a sporting event, prompting an emergency visit. The tubercle is tender, and the plain film shows irregularity and fragmentation of the distal tubercle (Fig. 6-8). A lateral film of the other side may be helpful, although Osgood-Schlatter disease often is unilateral. A knee immobilizer, ice, ibuprofen, crutches, and 48-h follow-up are the treatment for Osgood-Schlatter disease. Admission for open reduction and internal fixation (ORIF) is the treatment for the avulsion fracture.

Medial and Lateral Plateau Fractures

These are high-energy injuries involving both plateaus. There is much bleeding, ligamentous damage, and there may be popliteal vessel or tibial or peroneal nerve damage. Significant compartment syndrome risk is present.

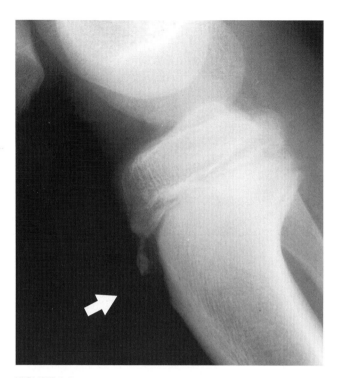

FIGURE 6-8

Osgood-Schlatter disease.

Intercondylar Eminence Fracture (Fig. 6-9)

The eminence, or tibial spine, is the attachment site of the anterior cruciate ligament (ACL). This is an ACL tear through bone. The patient usually can bear weight, although the knee may be locked in a flexed position. There will be a bloody effusion. The patient generally can go home with a knee immobilizer, ice, crutches, pain medicine, and follow-up in 48 h.

TESTS

Smaller fractures may need a computed tomographic (CT) scan to evaluate the exact degree of depression. Many orthopedists indicate surgery based on the number of millimeters of joint-line depression. The CT scan is good for this. It is not strictly an emergency test, but it may help to make a decision regarding admission.

Compartment syndrome should be kept in mind with plateau fractures. Extreme pain, pain with passive motion of the toes, tenseness of the leg, and elevated compartment pressure are the signs of compartment syndrome that should prompt surgical decompression before numbness and pulselessness develop (see Chap. 5)

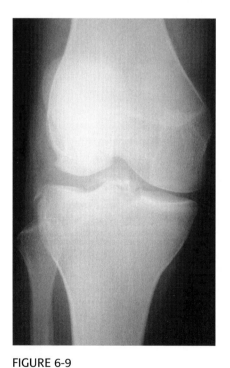
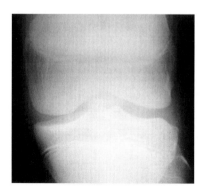
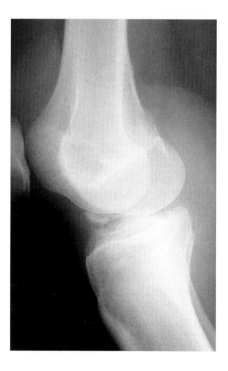

FIGURE 6-9

Intercondylar eminence fracture.

The perceived instability of the knee when there is a plateau fracture can suggest ligamentous damage, prompting an MRI study. It is usually the fracture that creates the instability, however. The MRI is truly useful when insufficiency fracture is suggested by tenderness of the upper tibia and pain with weightbearing.

TREATMENT

A knee immobilizer is essential. Even when you are admitting the patient, having the immobilizer on makes it less painful for the patient to move around in bed. It also prevents further displacement of the fracture. Lots of ice and two pillows under the knee, lengthwise, also help.

Most plateau fracture patients are admitted for surgery. A patient with an insufficiency fracture or a depression-type fracture of one plateau with less than 10 mm of depression on the plain film sometimes can go home, strictly non-weightbearing, with a knee immobilizer (and crutches or walker and narcotics) if the patient is strong enough. Warn the patient about compartment syndrome signs. Follow-up should be within 48 h.

SPECIAL CONCERNS

Aspiration of the knee with a tense effusion after trauma and a suspected insufficiency fracture is diagnostically helpful when the x-ray is negative. There is also some pain relief afforded by taking out effusion. Fat droplets in nearly pure blood are a sign that bone is broken. They look like the fat on top of chicken soup.

To aspirate the knee, first prep with Betadine and alcohol. Anesthetize the skin with 1 to 2 ml 1% lidocaine with a fine needle at the superolateral aspect of the patella. Then aspirate with an 18-gauge needle on a 60-ml syringe. Remember to connect the needle to the syringe loosely enough so that you can leave the needle in the knee and disconnect the syringe to empty it if you need to take out more than 60 ml. The effusion floats the patella—you want to slide the needle under the patella and aspirate slowly, rotating the needle so that it does not become clogged with synovium. Warn the patient that the fluid probably will come right back. Keep some pressure on the site with a gauze pad for 2 min after removing the needle. Finish with a bandage.

CHAPTER

7

Knee: Soft Tissues and Patella

NORMAL RADIOGRAPHS

- Anteroposterior (AP), lateral, and sunrise views (Fig. 7-1A–C)
- Bipartite patella (Fig. 7-2)

- Normal distance from tibia to patella on lateral view Fig. 7-3
- Arthritic changes (Fig. 7-4)
- Quadriceps tendon, patellar tendon, menisci, cruciates, collateral ligaments, and pes anserinus (Fig. 7-5)

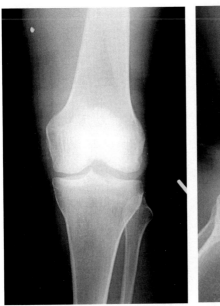
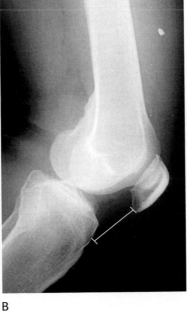
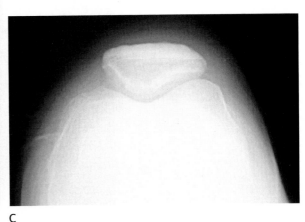

A
B
C

FIGURE 7-1

Normal knee. *A.* Anteroposterior (AP) view. *B.* Lateral view. *C.* Sunrise view.

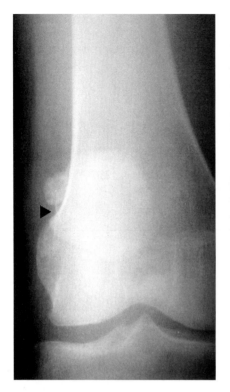

FIGURE 7-2

Bipartite patella (arrowhead).

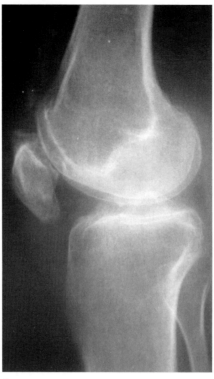

A

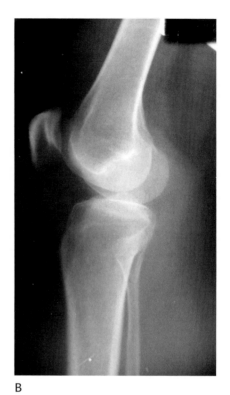

B

FIGURE 7-3

Lateral view with measurement of patella-tibial tubercle distance—*A.* baja *B.* alta.

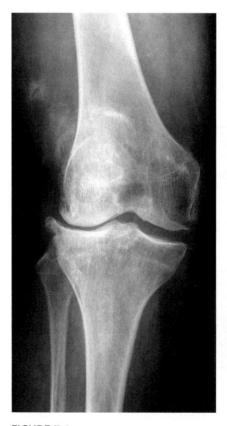

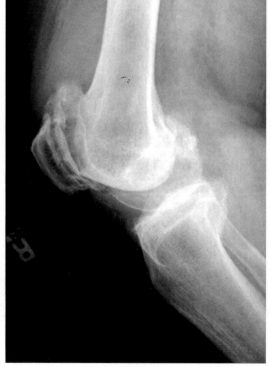

FIGURE 7-4

Arthritic knee.

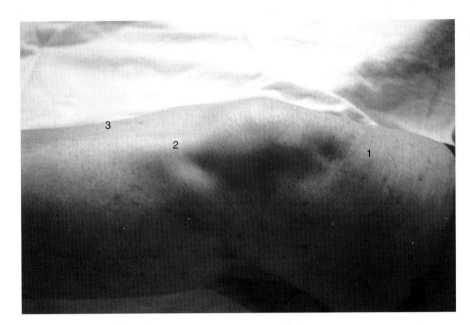

FIGURE 7-5

Quadriceps tendon (1), patellar tendon (2), pes anserinus (3).

PROBLEM LIST

Patella Fractures

- *Non-displaced* (Fig. 7-6). The plain film shows a patella fracture. This is either an avulsion, in which a thin shell or flake of bone is pulled away from the main body of the patella (usually from the distal tip), or a nondisplaced crack through the body. Hematomas can be large. The important clinical feature is that the patient is able, with pain, to do an active straight-leg raise. This means that the mechanical integrity of the extensor mechanism is being maintained by the soft tissues that envelop the patella. This patient generally can go home with a knee immobilizer, crutches, weightbearing as tolerated, and 48-h follow-up.

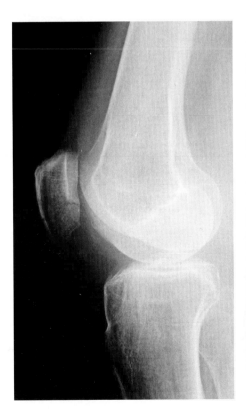
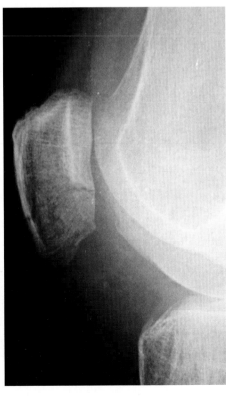

FIGURE 7-6

Patella fracture, nondisplaced.

FIGURE 7-7

Patella fracture, transverse, displaced.

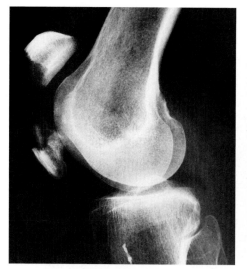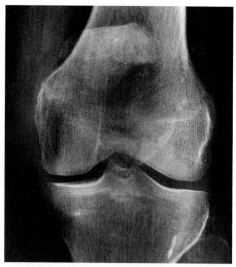

- *Transverse, displaced* (Fig. 7-7). Bone fails in tension. You often can feel the separation (a horizontal depression) in the midpatella. There is a large hematoma but often surprisingly little pain. The patient is unable to do an active straight-leg raise. The patient definitely needs an operation to repair the patella. If the patient is strong and reliable, he or she can go home with crutches and a knee immobilizer. Make it clear that the patient definitely requires surgery. Follow-up must be within 48 h. Most of these patients are admitted for next day surgery. Make sure that the immobilizer is on, either way.

- *Comminuted, displaced* (Fig. 7-8). This is a higher-energy injury with tension, as well as direct impact to the front of the knee. Generally, patients are in a good deal of pain and require admission for surgery. Do not forget to put on a knee immobilizer. Ice, elevation, and pain medicine also are necessary.

Rupture of the Infrapatellar Tendon

The patella may be higher than normal when viewed on lateral x-ray. Plain film also can be normal. A divot can be palpated with your thumb just distal to the

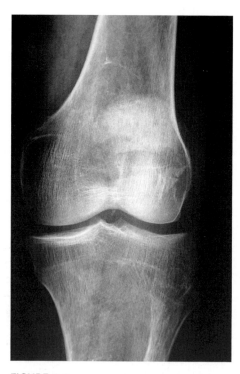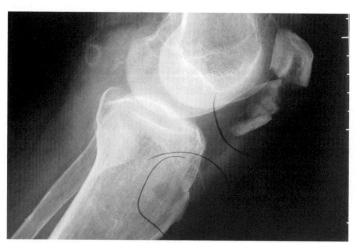

FIGURE 7-8

Patella fracture, comminuted, displaced.

distal tip of the patella. The patient is unable to do an active straight-leg raise. Pain is variable. Put on a knee immobilizer. Surgery is needed, so generally admit such patients, although a strong patient can go home for a day with crutches, weightbearing as tolerated, an immobilizer, and 24-h follow-up.

Rupture of the Quadriceps Tendon (Fig. 7-9)

This is a commonly missed injury. Retinacular tissues can hold the patella up in place, so the x-ray often is normal (i.e., the patella does not drop down as one would expect), and the large amount of generalized pain and swelling can lead to missing the cardinal sign on physical examination. This is a palpable divot just above the patella—a hole in the quadriceps tendon. The patient also will have difficulty performing an active straight-leg raise, although there are partial tears that, in a strong patient, do permit some straight-leg raising. Admit the patient for surgical repair in most instances. The strong patient, especially one with a partial tear, can go home with an immobilizer, crutches, weight-

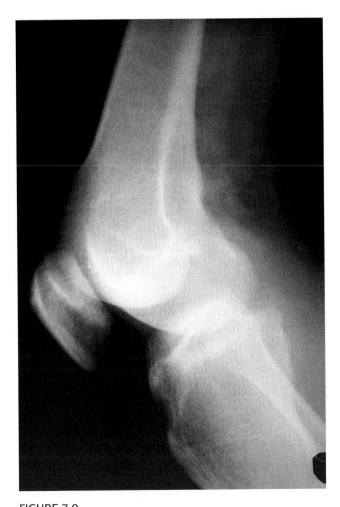

FIGURE 7-9

Quadriceps tendon rupture.

bearing as tolerated, and 24-h follow-up. These injuries get harder to repair as a result of muscle shortening, so admission generally is the best policy.

Ligament and Meniscal Injury

The plain film is normal, and the extensor mechanism is working (i.e., the patient can do an active straight-leg raise). There has been some trauma to the knee, and it hurts. This is a common emergency room presentation. Remember that if the knee examination is normal and the patient is skeletally immature, you may be looking at referred pain from the hip—so get an AP film of the pelvis looking for a slipped capital femoral epiphysis.

If there is tenderness about the knee with an effusion, there is likely an *internal derangement*—tear of meniscus, anterior cruciate ligament (ACL), or small articular surface fracture (see Chap. 6). Reproducible bony pain with bearing weight suggests a fracture. Mild effusion that develops within 3 h of injury suggests meniscal injury. Tense effusion that accumulates rapidly after hearing or feeling a "pop" suggests an ACL tear. ACL tears are quite common in athletic patients and skiers. An "x-ray classic" indicating an ACL rupture is Segond's or lateral capsular sign (Fig. 7-10). This is an avulsion of a tiny fleck of the lateral tibial margin caused by the same forces that rupture the ACL. Its presence pretty much confirms ACL injury, but Segond's sign itself is fairly uncommon even when the ACL is completely torn. Magnetic resonance imaging (MRI) eventually is necessary in nearly all these injuries.

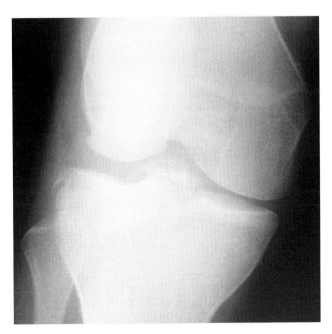

FIGURE 7-10

Segond's lateral capsular sign.

Atraumatic Painful Knee

Minimal or insignificant trauma in the history suggests a rheumatologic process. Pseudogout, which is an inflammatory diathesis associated with calcium pyrophosphate crystal deposition, is the most common of these. This knee shows osteoarthritic changes on plain film, it is warm, and the white blood cell count (WBC) and erythrocyte sedimentation rate (ESR) may be elevated. The ability to "see" the menisci on plain-film x-ray—because they are somewhat calcified—is a classic sign of pseudogout. It is not reliable, however. There is no wonder that many of these patients are admitted as septic arthritis patients.

True gout of the knee appears similarly. Most of these patients have had a gout attack previously and can tell you that this seems like another one. The serum urate concentration usually (but not always) is elevated here. Making a diagnosis based on microscopic crystal analysis is not easy. The crystals of urate or pyrophosphate on which you base the gout/pseudogout diagnosis can both dissolve in the joint fluid after aspiration. There can be a true septic arthritis with some crystals present incidentally. Every test can be normal or abnormal with infection, gout, rheumatoid disease, or pseudogout. What all this means is that you must phone the rheumatologist, internist, or as a last resort, the orthopedist and let him or her address these issues.

Septic arthritis of the knee, including Lyme disease, is one of the first things that comes to mind when a patient with an inflamed, atraumatic knee presents. Blood tests include a complete blood count (CBC), ESR, Lyme titer, and chemistry panel that includes urate. Emergency treatment must include an aspiration of the knee for culture and cell count before any antibiotic is given. Aspirating a knee that is full of fluid is easier than doing blood cultures. A dry knee is unlikely to be infected. Just prep the skin twice with Betadine and once with alcohol before putting the needle in. The lateral midpatellar area is a safe place to puncture, especially if you compress the site for 2 min after taking out the needle. Make sure you schedule the following tests.

KNEE ASPIRATE TESTS (ANY JOINT WITH SUSPICION OF INFECTION)

Cell count—put 2 ml in a CBC tube
Culture—aerobic, anaerobic, gonoccocal
Crystal analysis—red-top tube on ice
Gram stain
Lyme titer

Dislocation of the Knee (Fig. 7-11)

True dislocation of the knee is a surgical emergency that demands that you call for the orthopedist and the

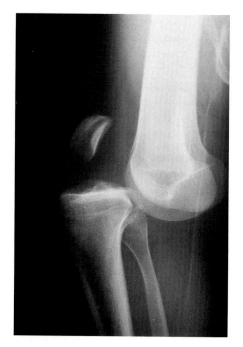

FIGURE 7-11

Dislocated knee.

vascular surgeon immediately. The risk of arterial and neurologic damage is very high. It must be borne in mind that the vast majority of knees that present with abnormal angulation have a fracture of the tibia or femur. So get the plain film before telling everyone that a dislocated knee just came in. A true dislocation will be apparent on the plain film—the tibia is not under the femur. There can be a dislocation that presents with normal films—reduced by the splint in transport. In this case you should get the history of dislocation from the emergency medical technicians.

When there is a true dislocation, you will find complete loss of ligamentous stability, i.e., a floppy knee, that is tense with bloody effusion and severe pain. The presence or absence of pulses in the foot must be documented, and the knee must be immobilized in the position in which it arrived. Start an IV, and get the patient ready for the operating room. Remember that this is not a subtle injury. Every ligament and the capsule of the knee are torn. Arteries are torn. Do not reduce this until both services (orthopedics and vascular surgery) are present—and then let them do it. This is, fortunately, fairly uncommon.

Dislocation of the Patella (Fig. 7-12)

This is a common injury in adolescent girls. It is almost invariably what a patient refers to when they tell you, "I dislocated my knee, but it went back into

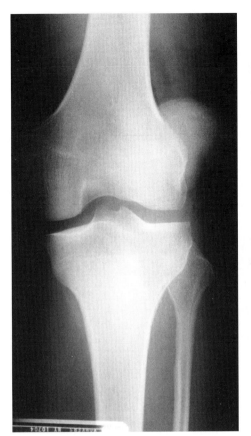

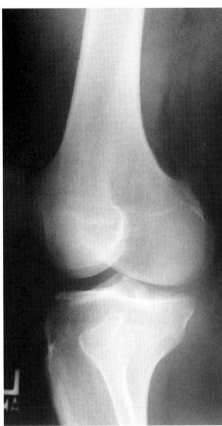

FIGURE 7-12

Dislocated patella.

place." It occurs as the patient is getting up from a deep squat or from sitting on the floor. The patella jumps out of the trochlea and goes laterally. The patient occasionally will get to the emergency room with the patella still dislocated. This patient is in a lot of pain with the knee locked in mild flexion. The anterior aspect of the knee feels sharp—there is no patella there. The plain film shows that the patella is off to the side.

This is a very easy dislocation to reduce. You need only straighten out the knee, sometimes giving a slight medial push to the patella. Muscle spasm and voluntary splinting are the only things preventing extension and reduction. So give the patient some narcotic and benzodiazepine, if necessary. Calm the patient down, place the patient supine, and lift the leg, gently, by the ankle. When the patella reduces, get a plain film to document reduction, put on a knee immobilizer, and send the patient home with ice, crutches, and 48-h orthopedic follow-up.

More commonly, the patella dislocation was reduced before the patient got to the emergency room. The history, a normal plain film, valgus knees, and tenderness around the patella with otherwise good knee

function confirm this diagnosis. Give this patient a knee immobilizer and cane with orthopedic follow-up within 4 days.

TESTS

MRI of the knee is a great way to verify all the injuries in this section. It is only essential to the diagnosis of pure soft tissue injuries, however. The need for MRI in the emergency setting is debatable. Few initial management decisions hinge on MRI findings. Patients nevertheless expect more and more convenience and "consumer satisfaction" in medical care. Their athletic careers, even in grammar school, are ever more important. Orthopedists love to take in new patients with their workup already done, diagnosis secured, and no health maintenance organization (HMO) test-justifying letters to write. Coupled with the healthy profits that most hospitals realize from MRI, this has meant more "emergency" MRI studies of acute knee injuries.

Overall, you will not be faulted for getting an MRI unless a clear fracture is present on plain film. Just don't let the availability of the MRI put your diagnostic zeal to sleep.

C H A P T E R

8

Knee: Distal Femur

NORMAL RADIOGRAPHS

- Anteroposterior (AP) view of distal femur/knee (Fig. 8-1A)
- Lateral view of distal femur/knee (Fig. 8-1B)

Metaphysis, diaphysis of femur
Medial, lateral condyles
Trochlea

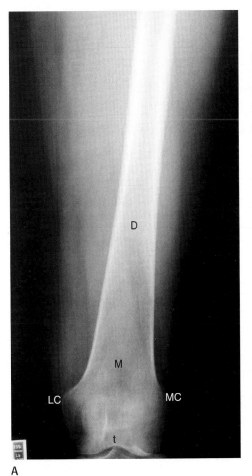

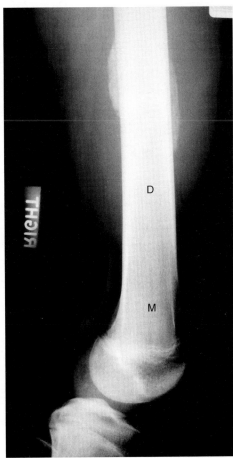

A

B

FIGURE 8-1

Normal knee, distal femur. *A.* Anteroposterior (AP) view. *B.* Lateral view. M = metaphysis; D = diaphysis of femur; MC = medial; LC = lateral condyles; t = trochlea. Note old heterotropic ossification (myositis ossificans) on lateral view (•).

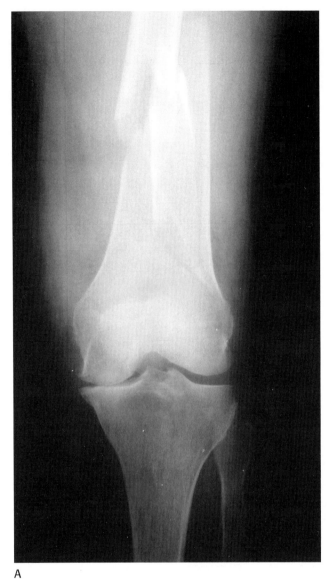
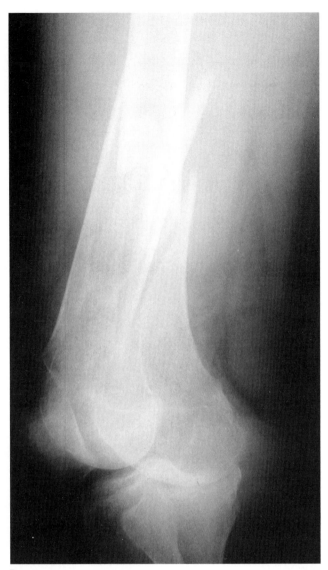

A   B

FIGURE 8-2

Supracondylar fracture. *A.* Anteroposterior (AP) view. *B.* Lateral view.

PROBLEM LIST

Supracondylar Fracture (Fig. 8-2*A*, *B*)

This is a fracture within the metaphyseal flare of the distal femur. Much swelling, pain, and angular deformity are common. Bleeding from the bone surfaces and surrounding tissues can be severe—so start intravenous (IV) fluids and send for laboratory tests, apply ice, and order narcotics. Damage to the nearby popliteal blood vessels or the tibial and peroneal nerves is also associated. Good documentation of the neurocirculatory status of the affected side is a must.

These fractures are always unstable, even if nondisplaced. Patients must be immobilized and admitted.

Use straight traction on the leg to get the limb straight enough to put on a knee immobilizer. Call the orthopedist as soon as the plain films are ready.

Intercondylar Fracture (Fig. 8-3)

This is a fracture of the distal femur that breaks into the articular surface of the knee. There is often a supracondylar component that goes up into the metaphyseal flare. Such fractures are essentially a subset of supracondylar fractures that are somewhat harder to fix. In the emergency room, such patients require a knee immobilizer, ice, elevation, neurocirculatory checks, narcotics, IV fluid, admission, and a call to the orthopedist.

FIGURE 8-3

A. Transverse Supracondylar fracture
B. medial condylar fracture
C. shaft fracture with intercondylar extension.

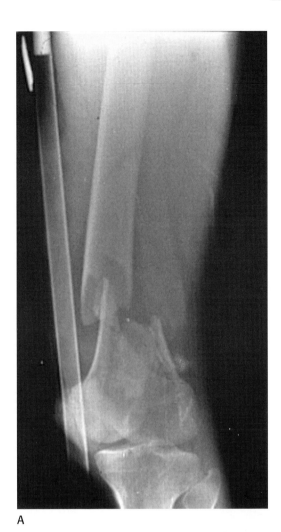

A

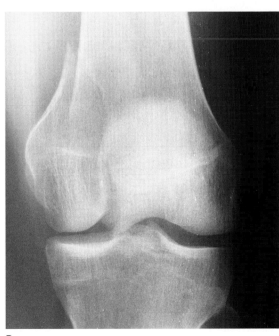

B

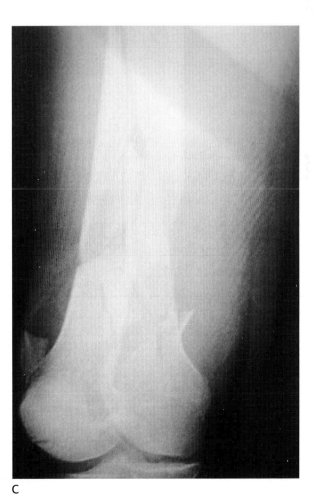

C

9

Femoral Shaft

NORMAL RADIOGRAPHS

- Anteroposterior (AP) and lateral plain films of the femur (Fig. 9-1*A*, *B*)

PROBLEM LIST

Fractures are termed *shaft fractures* when they involve primarily the femoral diaphysis. There is no clear distinction; thus the term *femoral shaft fracture* can be used for a high supracondylar fracture that goes up from the metaphysis into the diaphysis or for a low subtrochanteric fracture that extends down from the area of the lesser trochanter. There is no clear distinction between a high shaft fracture and a low subtroch fracture.

The person to whom you are describing the fracture will be interested in whether it is a straight, transverse fracture (Fig. 9-2) or a long and oblique fracture (Fig. 9-3). The degree of comminution (how many pieces) is also important to the definitive orthopedic management.

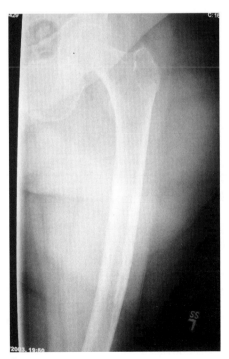

A

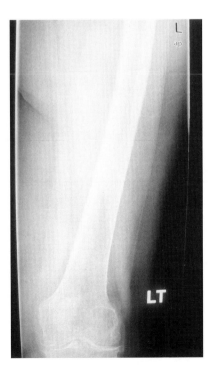

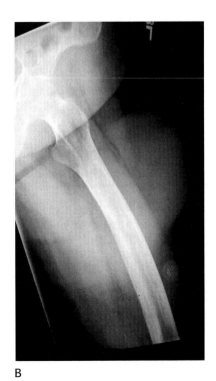

B

FIGURE 9-1

Femur shaft, normal. *A.* Anteroposterior (AP) view. *B.* Lateral view.

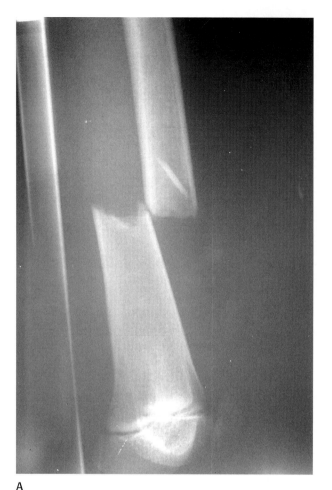

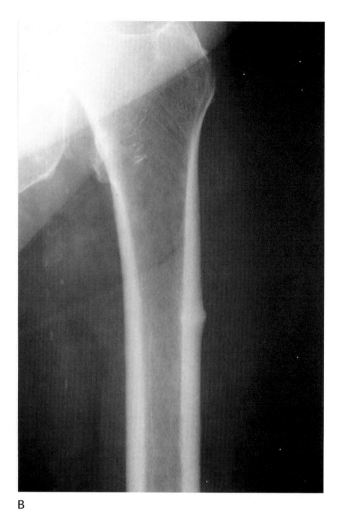

A   B

FIGURE 9-2

A. Transverse fractures of the femoral shaft. *B.* Incomplete or stress fracture of femoral shaft.

TREATMENT

All such patients are admitted. Intravenous (IV) fluids, pain medication, ice to the fracture site, and neurocirculatory checks are recommended. These fractures are often the result of serious trauma, so send for laboratory tests and check the rest of the patient for head, spine, and visceral injuries. A Foley catheter is often a good idea. Call in the orthopedist as soon as you make the diagnosis.

SPECIAL CONCERNS

Compartment syndrome of the thigh is rare but can occur. Consider it if pain is increasing intolerable.

Myoglobinemia causing renal damage can occur due to muscle damage in the thigh. The low-flow state associated with blood loss and hypovolemia increases the risk. Adequate hydration and Foley catheter placement are good procedures to follow. Check with whomever will be managing the patient medically before alkalinizing the urine. This is done rarely.

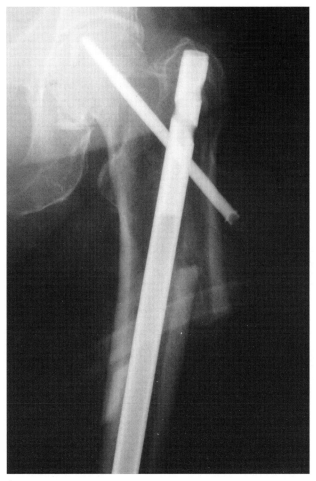

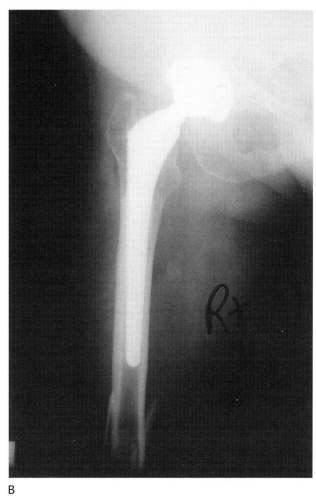

A   B

FIGURE 9-3

Oblique fractures of the femoral shaft. *A.* with internal fixation in place. *B.* Below prosthetic hip stem.

10

Hip and Proximal Femur

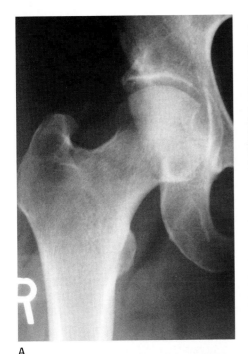

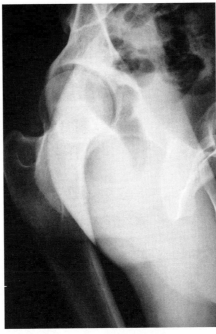

A

B

NORMAL RADIOGRAPHS

- Anteroposterior (AP) and lateral radiographs of normal hip (Fig. 10-1*A*, *B*)
- Cemented bipolar hemiarthroplasty in AP and lateral projection (Fig. 10-1*C*, *D*)

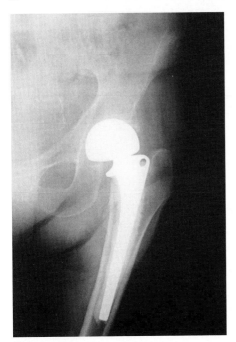

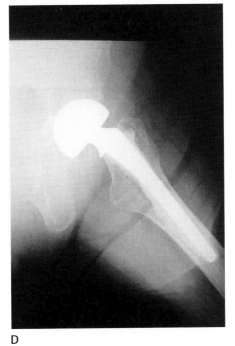

C

D

FIGURE 10-1

Normal hip. *A.* AP view. *B.* Lateral view. Replaced hip (Bipolar hemiarthroplasty). *C.* AP view. *D.* Lateral view.

FIGURE 10-2

A. Normal male pelvis. *B.* Pelvis with moderate osteoarthritis of right hip and lumbar spine – no fractures. *C.* Pelvis status post open reduction, internal fixation of right hip with Haig Nail. Fracture is healed. *D.* Pelvis status post right total hip replacement. Osteitis pubis condensans and left hip osteoarthritis are present.

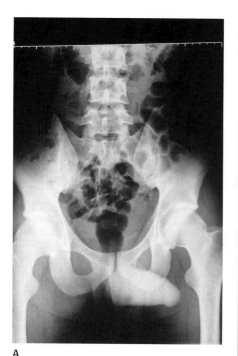

A

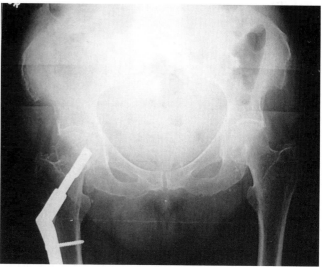

C

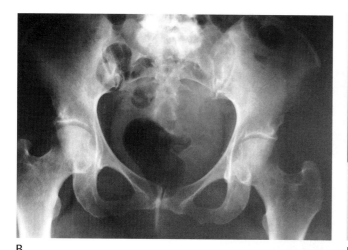

B

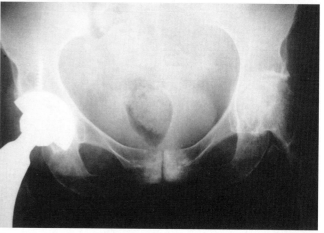

D

FIGURE 10-3

Oblique photograph of model pelvis.

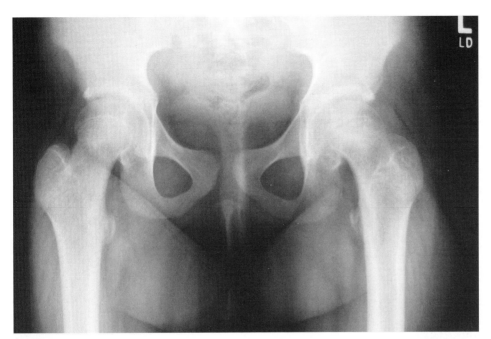

A

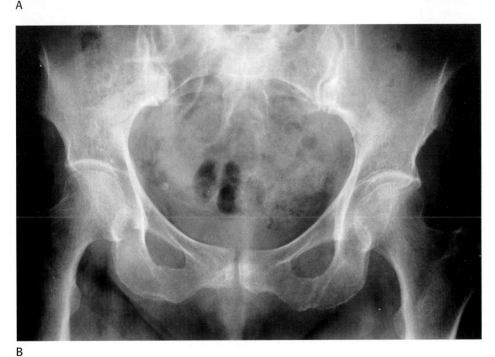

B

FIGURE 10-4

A. Normal hips. *B.* Osteopenic hips.

• Well-mineralized versus osteopenic hip (Fig. 10-4*A, B*)

PROBLEM LIST

The most important fractures of the hip fall into three anatomic categories.

• *Subtrochanteric* (Fig. 10-5). These primarily involve the hard cortical bone below the lesser trochanter. They may extend up slightly into the intertrochanteric zone or down into the femoral shaft.

• *Intertrochanteric* (Fig. 10-6*A–C*). These primarily involve the well-vascularized cancellous bone of the intertrochanteric zone. You will hear the term *basicervical* applied to some fractures. These are true intertrochanteric fractures. The basicervical region is the base of the femoral neck anatomically, but it is outside the hip capsule and so has a good blood supply from both sides of the fracture. Intertrochanteric fractures heal reliably when fixed internally.

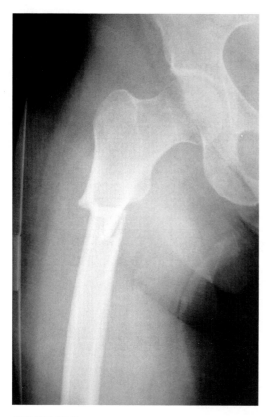

FIGURE 10-5

Subtrochanteric fracture.

FIGURE 10-6

Intertrochanteric hip fracture. *A.* Grade 1. *B.* Grade 2. *C.* Grade 3.

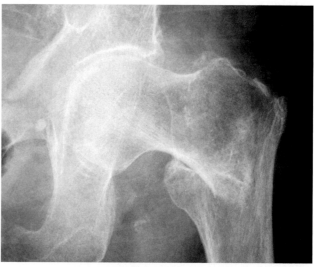

A

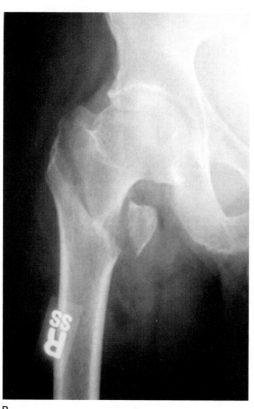

B

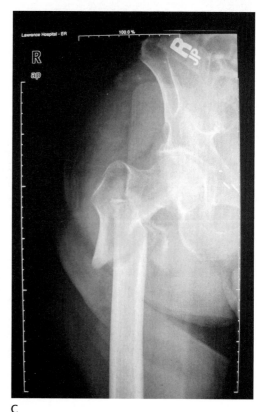

C

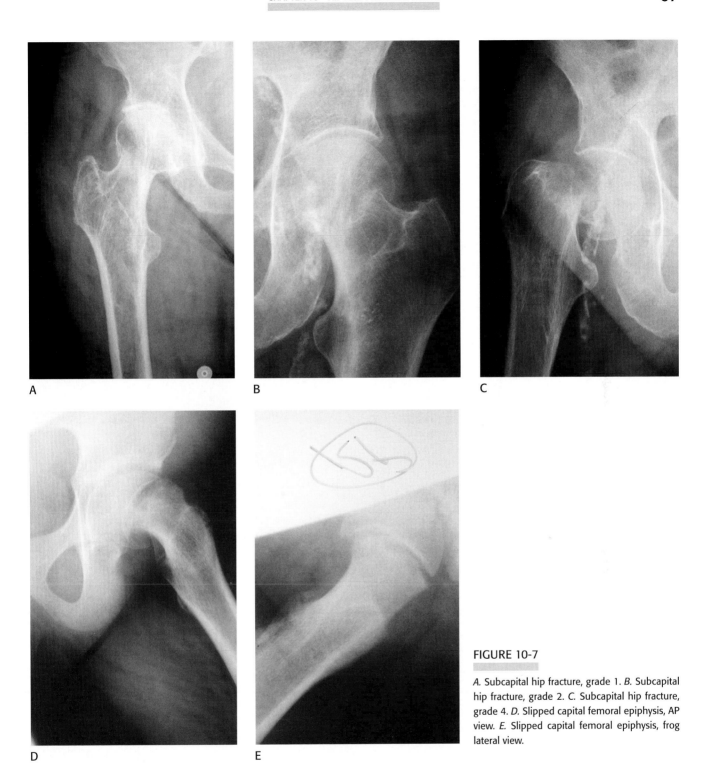

FIGURE 10-7

A. Subcapital hip fracture, grade 1. *B.* Subcapital hip fracture, grade 2. *C.* Subcapital hip fracture, grade 4. *D.* Slipped capital femoral epiphysis, AP view. *E.* Slipped capital femoral epiphysis, frog lateral view.

- *Subcapital* (Fig. 10-7*A–E*). These include fractures of the femoral neck, the femoral head, and the subcapital region, which is an unfortunate bit of orthopedic terminology meaning "the femoral neck, definitely within the capsule" (in contradistinction to the basicervical region which is "femoral neck, probably outside the capsule"). Fractures here may need to be treated with prosthetic replacement of the femoral head.

  Fractures of the true femoral head can occur. They often are associated with dislocation of the natural hip. Femoral head fractures without dislocation generally are treated like femoral neck fractures.

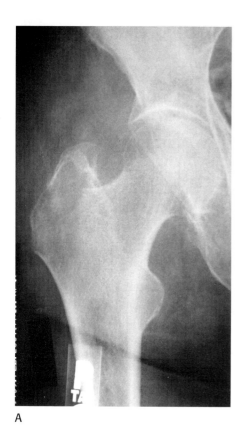

A

FIGURE 10-8

A. Fracture, greater trochanter—plain film. *B.* Magnetic resonance imaging (MRI).

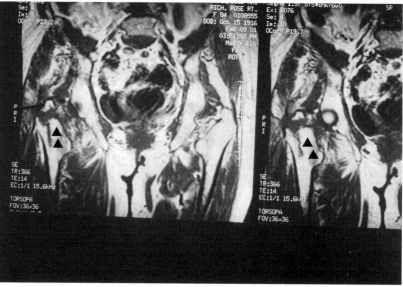

B

Greater Trochanteric Fractures (Fig. 10-8)

If only the greater trochanter has fractured, the weight-bearing axis is intact, and although in pain, this patient may bear weight without danger. These fractures hurt a lot, and because the attachment of the hip abductors is broken off, these fractures may produce a limp for up to a year. Nevertheless, these fractures are hardly ever treated surgically because the nonsurgical results are very good. Most patients are admitted for in-hospital physical therapy and pain control.

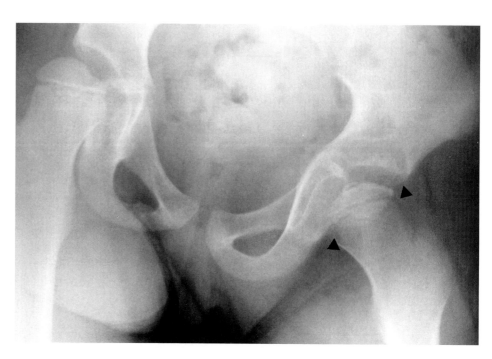

FIGURE 10-9

Perthes disease of left hip.

Slipped Capital Femoral Epiphysis (SCFE) (see Fig. 10-7D)

Called a "skiffee" by most orthopedists, this is essentially a Salter I subcapital fracture of the hip. It is common in 10- to 16-year-olds with or without trauma, and although this is a hip problem, it commonly produces only knee pain as a symptom—so get an AP view of the pelvis on every child in this age range who complains of knee pain but has a negative or equivocal knee examination. The epiphysis that includes the actual head of the femur slides posteroinferiorly as the cartilaginous growth plate (the physis) fails in shear. SCFE is generally treated with internal fixation, and so it must be recognized and the patient admitted. The lower grades of SCFE can only be seen on lateral films, so be sure to order a frog lateral pelvis view (see Fig. 10-7E), as well as the standard AP pelvic view when hip or knee pain is the complaint in a young teen.

Perthes Disease

An idiopathic avascular necrosis of the femoral head occurring in children, Perthes disease is not a common emergency presentation but often has a dramatic radiographic appearance (Fig. 10-9). Generally treated by specialized pediatric orthopedists, crutches to limit weightbearing, and mild pain medication are appro-priate in the emergency setting, with pediatric orthopedic follow-up in 48 h.

RADIOGRAPHIC CATEGORIES

Hip fractures can be obviously displaced on plain-film x-rays, undisplaced but still visible on plain-film x-rays, or undisplaced and visible only on magnetic resonance imaging (MRI). This last category is fairly new, but it is the reason why an emergency MRI of the hip is now indicated for patients with clear signs of hip fracture but a negative plain film.

These "MRI fractures" are important because they can be fixed internally with two small screws inserted through an inch-long incision under local anesthesia. If the fracture is not detected and the patient walks on the hip, there is a good chance of the fracture displacing, in which case a much larger operation with significantly greater morbidity becomes necessary.

HIP DISLOCATIONS

Dislocations of Prosthetic Hips (Fig. 10-10)

These are by far the most common. There are two types of prostheses: total-hip prostheses, in which the artificial

FIGURE 10-10

Dislocated total-hip arthroplasty.

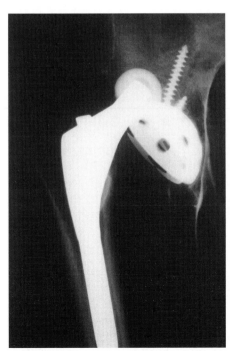

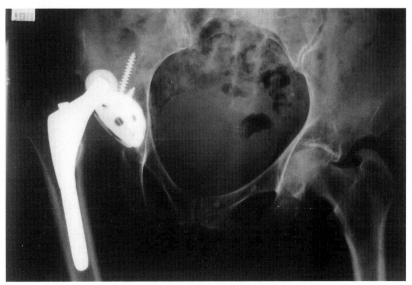

A

B

FIGURE 10-11

Dislocated natural hip.

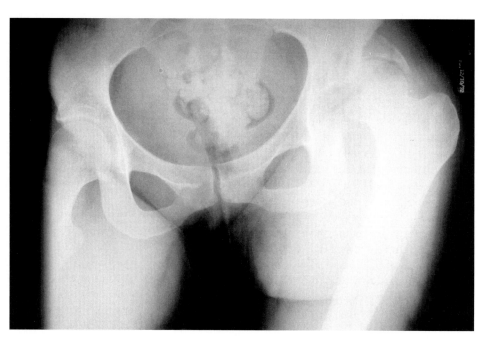

acetabular resurfacing component is fixed within the bony acetabulum, and hemiarthroplasties, in which a large metallic ball is placed directly into the bony acetabulum, which is not resurfaced. Both of these can dislocate—meaning that the prosthetic ball comes out of socket. The dislocated total hip usually can be reduced nonsurgically, as can the simple unipolar hemiarthoplasty, which is a large, solid metal ball on a stem (the Austin-Moore is the classic model). Bipolar hemiarthroplasties (see Fig. 10-1C, D) that dislocate usually cannot be reduced without being exposed surgically. These have a "ball within a ball" design.

Dislocations of Natural Hips (Fig. 10-11)

These are high-energy injuries, usually involving vehicular trauma or contact sports. There are chronic congenital dislocations that are not emergencies but which may be noted incidentally.

TREATMENT

All acute hip fractures require hospital admission and bed rest. Put the leg of the affected side on a pillow, use pain medication as needed, start intravenous (IV) fluids, and call the orthopedist and the medical doctor. Same day surgery is becoming common for hip fractures, so do not feed these patients until it is clear that surgery will not be done for at least 8 h.

A complete blood count (CBC), blood chemistries, an electrocardiogram (ECG), a chest film, and urinalysis (UA) are standard admission tests for hip patients. Clotting parameters, blood gases, and a clot to the

blood bank are useful as well. Palpate the iliac spines, the pubic rami, and the sacrum during your examination. (See Fig. 10-3 to keep in mind the shape of the pelvic structures you are examining.) Quite a few pubic ramus and sacral fractures go unnoticed when we are mesmerized by the fractured hip.

Hip dislocations need to be reduced as soon as possible. The orthopedist generally has to help with these—they are among the most difficult reductions in terms of the shear physical strength required. You may be asked if the hip is "out the back" (dislocated posterior) or "out the front" (dislocated anterior). The most reliable answer to this is to say that it's probably posterior if the lower extremity is rotated internally and probably anterior if it is rotated externally. A good deal of IV sedation is needed to reduce a dislocated hip. General anesthesia is often necessary.

A true medical emergency exists in the case of a dislocated natural hip because every hour the femoral head stays out of the acetabulum increases the likelihood of avascular necrosis of the head. A dislocated prosthetic hip is not quite as urgent but should be reduced as soon as possible (within 12 h).

Sciatic nerve injury is possible with hip fractures and dislocations. Be sure to document the patient's strength of dorsiflexion of the ankle and toes on the affected side.

TESTS

As mentioned earlier, when a patient clinically seems to have a hip fracture but there is no fracture visible on x-ray, an MRI of the hip is useful (see Fig. 10-8). The physical examination in these cases of nondisplaced, unvisualized hip fracture is remarkable for reproducible hip pain (deep to the greater trochanter or in the groin) that increases with load or internal/external rotation of the hip.

A good bit of judgment goes into making the decision to send the patient for emergency MRI. The factor that perhaps plays the largest role is whether or not the patient is able to go home. Remember that a patient who is unable to walk because of hip pain probably has to be admitted. The MRI can be done on an inpatient basis in this case. The MRI becomes a part of your emergency workup when the decision to admit hinges on it.

When there has been some trauma and there is true hip pain, get AP, lateral, and internal rotation views of the hip, as well as an AP view of the pelvis. If there are no pelvic or hip fractures on careful reading of these films and the patient can get around well enough with a walker or crutches, nothing but a clear reading on MRI permits you to send that patient home secure in the knowledge that he or she will not be rolling back in with a displaced hip fracture later in the week.

Bone scans are sensitive tests for fracture, but they require up to 72 h after injury to become positive (more in very old or very sick patients). They are used rarely in the emergency setting.

CHAPTER

11

Pelvis, Acetabulum, Sacrum, and Coccyx

NORMAL RADIOGRAPHS

Figure 11-1A is an anteroposterior (AP) view of the pelvis showing pubic rami, ischial rami, iliac wings, acetabulum, tear-drop, symphysis, sacrum, coccyx, sacroiliac joint, and quadrilateral surface. Figure 11-1B is an AP view of a younger patient's pelvis with the same labels.

Three bones form the pelvis: the ischium, which you sit on; the ilium, which you are touching when you put your hands "on your hips"; and the pubis, which is palpable in the groin. They come together at the acetabulum. The sacrum is the strong shield-shaped bone at the base of the spine that fits in between the two huge iliac wings posteriorly.

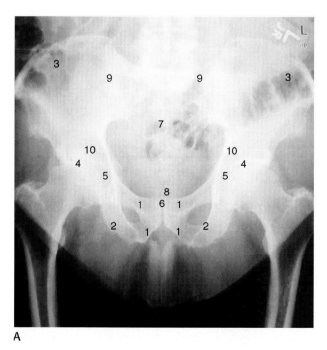

A

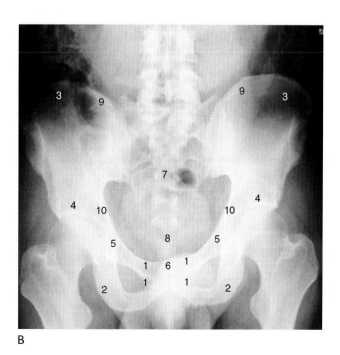

B

FIGURE 11-1

A. Normal pelvis, AP view. *B.* Model of pelvis. (1) pubic ramus (2) ischial ramus (3) iliac wing (4) acetabulum (5) tear drop (6) symphysis pubis (7) sacrum (8) coccyx (9) sacroiliac joint (10) quadrilateral surface.

PROBLEM LIST

Who gets an AP pelvic film? Almost everybody, including patients

- With pelvic pain after a fall or other trauma
- With low back pain
- With hip pain
- With thigh pain
- Who are old or noncommunicative and who have had trauma and do not walk
- Who are old or noncommunicative and who have trauma and an unexplained fall in hematocrit

- With every kind of high-speed trauma
- Who have been injured in any kind of jump

This is to say: *Be liberal in ordering this film.* You will pick up pelvic, sacral, and hip fractures that otherwise would be missed.

MINOR PELVIC FRACTURES

Pubic ramus fractures (Fig. 11-2). Sometimes these are hard to see on plain films. However, they are quite common causes of groin and hip pain after trauma in

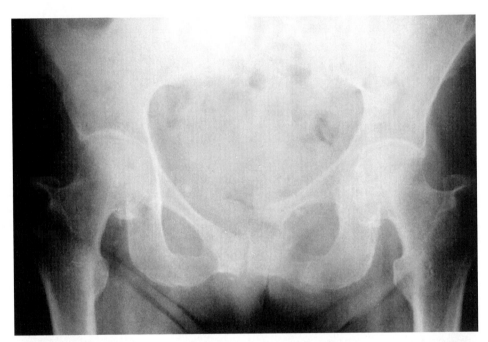

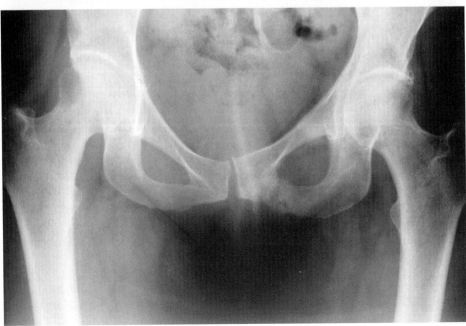

FIGURE 11-2

Pubic ramus fracture.

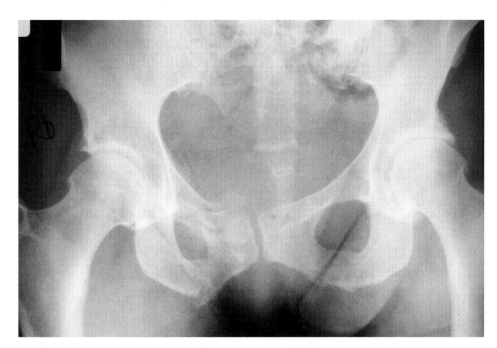

FIGURE 11-3

Ischial ramus fractures as well as pubic ramus.

young people. They are more common and can be spontaneous in older people (truly minimal trauma). Always check for tenderness of the bony pubic rami in anyone with hip/groin pain. Pubic ramus fractures accompany hip fractures in many patients. Look for one when you see the other.

Ischial ramus fractures (Fig. 11-3). Note that pubic fractures are also present. Often these are even harder to detect because of the way the ischium curves upward and forward as it flows into the pubis. As with pubic fractures, there is pain and tenderness. An avul-

sion of a chunk of the ischium by violent use of the hamstring muscles is seen in hurdlers. Treat with crutches, weightbearing as tolerated, and 48-h follow-up.

Iliac wing fractures (Fig. 11-4). These are higher-energy injuries—usually a fall at speed or vehicular trauma with direct force to the pelvis. There is a folding down or up of the wide, flat iliac bone. There is much pain with lateral compression of the pelvis. Patients also can have a large retroperitoneal or even an anterior abdominal hematoma.

FIGURE 11-4

Iliac wing fracture: (*A*) iliac wing fracture; (*B*) avulsion fracture of superior acetabular lip.

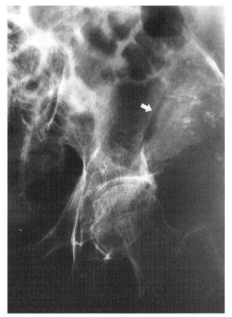

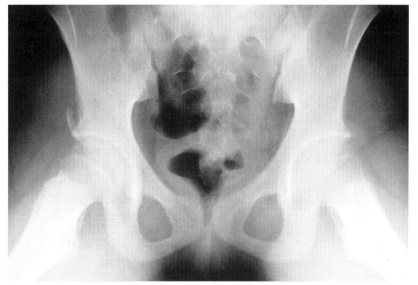

A B

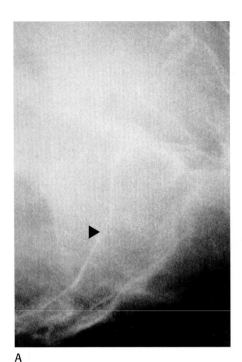

A

FIGURE 11-5

Sacral fractures. *A.* lateral view *B.* AP view.

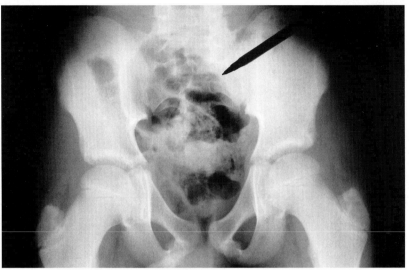

B

- *Sacral fractures* (Fig. 11-5). These can be included with minor pelvic fractures. History of a fall and local pain with sitting are the historical clues. These generally are diagnosed in the emergency room by reproducible local tenderness on the sacrum and an x-ray showing a "possible sacral fracture." They are hard to see on plain films. Order special sacral views if the patient has pain and tenderness below the belt line. Magnetic resonance imaging (MRI) or a computed tomographic (CT) scan is the best way to secure this diagnosis, but since there is no real change in emergency room management if the diagnosis is secured, you can leave it to the orthopedist to get these tests on an elective basis.
- *Acetabular fractures* (Fig. 11-6A–C). Figure 11-6E is an oblique Judet view clearly showing a fracture of the anterior column or iliac portion of the acetabulum. Minimal or moderate displacement (<1 cm) acetabular fractures are treated like other

minor pelvic fractures. Check the contour of the quadrilateral surface and compare it with the unaffected side to make the diagnosis on plain fim. Get Judet views (Fig. 11-7) for improved visualization of the acetabular contours. Admit these patients and place them on bed rest.

MINOR PELVIC FRACTURES: TREATMENT

Although these fractures do not generally require surgery, patients are often admitted for pain control, hematocrit monitoring (they can bleed quite a bit), and deep vein thrombosis (DVT) prophylaxis (DVT is common). Call the orthopedist and the internist to discuss admission. In the emergency room, the important issues are blood count, ruling out genitourinary damage, and analgesia. If these patients are to go home, self-care issues predominate. These must be sorted out before discharge from the emergency room.

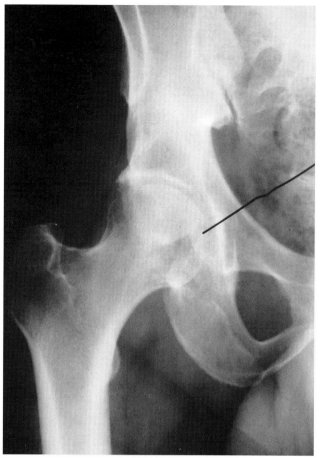

A

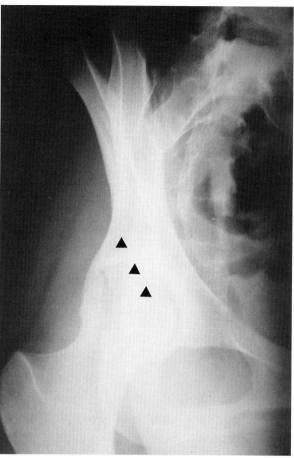

B

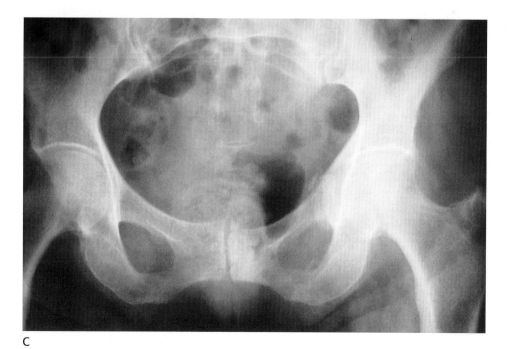

C

FIGURE 11-6

Acetabular fracture. *A.* Posterior column acetabular fracture – from ischium into acetabulum AP view *B.* Posterior lip acetabular fracture (arrowheads) *C.* Protusio acetabuli – central fracture of acetabular dome.

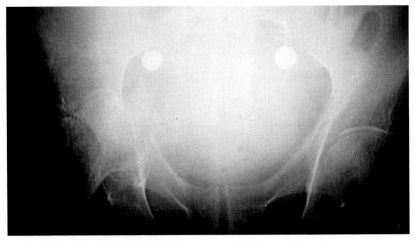

D

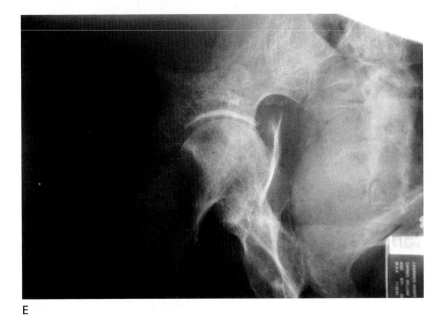

E

FIGURE 11-6

Acetabular fracture. *D*. Anterior column acetabular fracture seen on AP view of pelvis *E*. Same fracture in *D*. seen more clearly on iliac oblique Judet view.

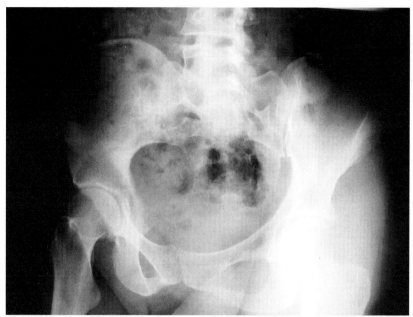

A

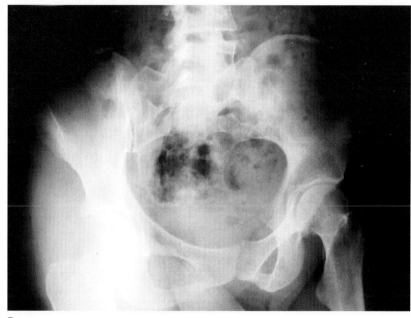

B

FIGURE 11-7

Judet view. *A.* Obturator oblique, injured side tilted up 45°. *B.* Iliac oblique, injured side tilted down 45°.

TESTS

CT scans of the pelvis give excellent fracture definition. You can get pelvic inlet and outlet films in the emergency room if the fractures are difficult to see on the AP pelvic film. Urinalysis (UA) and serial complete blood counts (CBCs) are in order for most pelvic fractures.

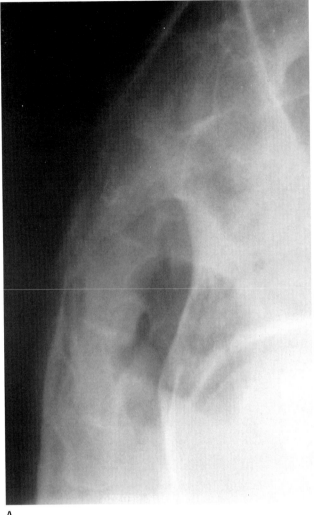

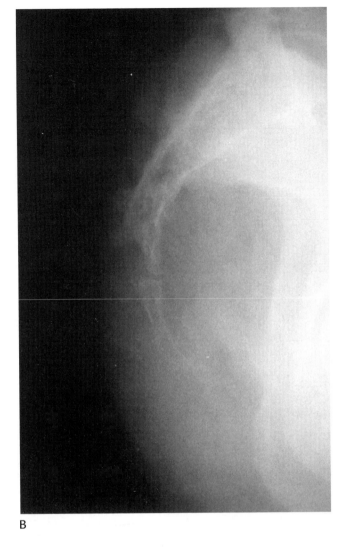

A

B

FIGURE 11-8

Coccyx fractures.

COCCYX FRACTURES (FIG. 11-8)

Classically, these result from a fall "on the bottom." Most patients volunteer that they think they have broken their "tail bone." The lateral film of the coccyx may show a clearcut fracture; it usually just shows that the last coccygeal segments are "bent" forward. Do a gentle rectal examination if there is worry about injury there (rare). Send the patient home with plenty of narcotic and a stool softener. Instruct the patient to "stay off it"—sit on one haunch. Follow-up is necessary within a week.

MAJOR PELVIC FRACTURES

These are much less common but are far from rare. There are many patterns, but the key feature is that two displaced breaks are present in the pelvic "ring" and there is gross distortion of the pelvis—one entire side can be higher than the other (the Malgaigne or vertical shear pattern; Fig. 11-9) or the halves of the pelvis are splayed apart (the diastasis or the "open book" pattern; Fig. 11-10).

The "open book" pattern may occur without obvious fracture, just wide separation of the pubic symphysis

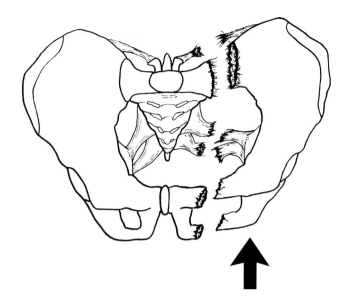

◄ FIGURE 11-9

Vertical shear fracture of pelvis, Malgaigne type.

(>4 cm), with the iliac wings hinging on the sacroiliac ligaments. Bladder and urethral injury, in addition to blood loss, can be present here. Any blood at the urethral meatus means that a retrograde urethrogram should be performed before placing a urinary catheter, and the catheter should be placed very gingerly even if the urethrogram is normal. Call in the urologist for any suggestion of bladder or urethral trauma.

Dislocation of the sacroiliac joint; large, displaced fractures through the sacrum; and large, displaced fractures into the acetabulum all qualify as major pelvic fractures. The great amount of internal bleeding

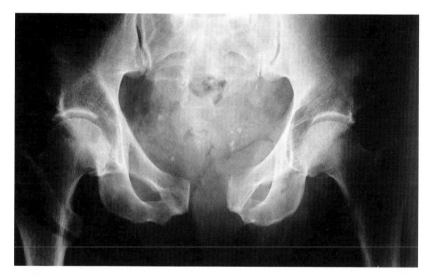

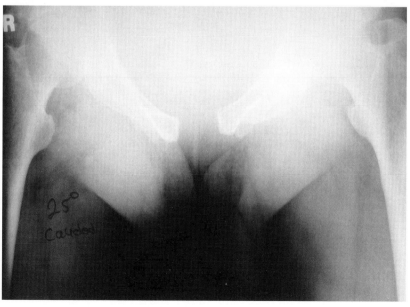

FIGURE 11-10

Pelvic diastasis injuries, "open book" type.

from these fractures often can be stopped only by emergency surgical fixation. You cannot splint a pelvic fracture. The important job for the emergency physician is to recognize the fracture and associated abdominal and genitourinary trauma; call the trauma, orthopedics, and urology services; and support the patient hemodynamically. There are hospitals from which transfer to a trauma center is the best treatment for these patients. Have the orthopedist or traumatologist on call sort this out and arrange it.

High-energy trauma produces these fractures. Internal bleeding from bone and adjacent soft tissues is often severe. These are true surgical emergencies; the internal or external fixation that the orthopedist applies is able to slow or stop the bleeding in many cases. Send for laboratory tests and type and crossmatch blood as soon as the diagnosis is made. Check for genitourinary trauma. Record the neurologic and vascular examinations of the lower extremities. Do a retrograde urethrogram if there is blood at the penile or urethral meatus. Start intravenous (IV) fluids, and be sure to recheck the hematocrit as it equilibrates (within 2 h). Call in orthopedics and a surgical traumatologist immediately.

12

Fingers: The Phalanges

NORMAL RADIOGRAPHS

Figure 12-1 contains anteroposterior (AP), lateral, and oblique radiographs of the hand showing the proximal, middle, and distal phalanges. Remember, the thumb has no middle phalanx. The common terminology referes to the DIP (dee.eye.pee) PIP and MP joints of the thumb, index, long, ring and little fingers. No one is quite sure what the 'middle joint of the second finger' means. See the labels in Fig. 12. The level of the MP joints is more proximal than most people think when looked at on the volar surface (the palm) of the hand. The palmar flexion crease marks the MP joint line. See this in Fig 12-2. Note that the location of MP joint is more proximal than the web space. A flexion crease marks the MP joint on the volar side. Figure 12-3 is a lateral film of the finger showing the fingernail. See also Figs. 12-4 through 12-6.

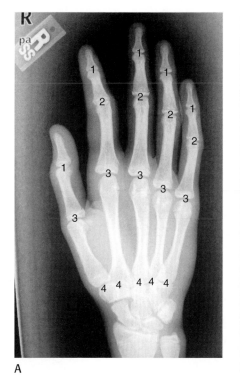

A

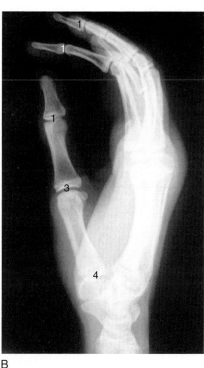

B

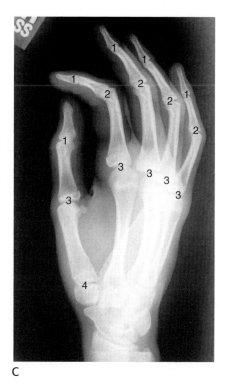

C

FIGURE 12-1

Normal hand. *A.* AP view. *B.* Lateral view. *C.* Oblique view. (1) DIP = distal interphalangeal (2) PIP = proximal interphalangeal (3) MP = metacarpophalangeal (4) CMC = carpometacarpal.

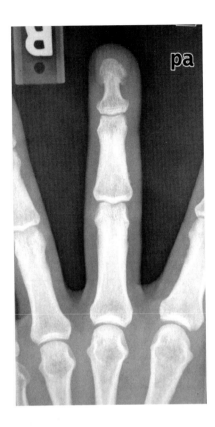

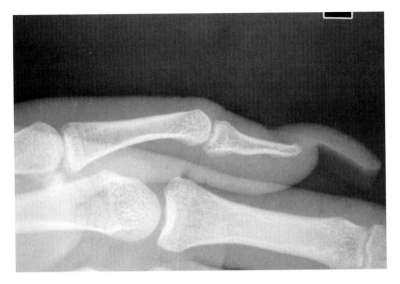

FIGURE 12-3

Lateral view of a fingernail.

FIGURE 12-2

Radiograph with soft-tissue technique shows relationship of skin landmarks to underlying joints. The MP joints are at the level of the palmar flexion crease. The fingernail covers half the distal phalanx.

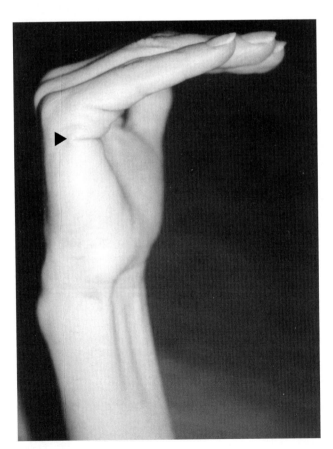

FIGURE 12-4

Intrinsic plus position (DIP flexion = deep flexor function). Arrowhead marks the palmar flexion crease/MP joint level.

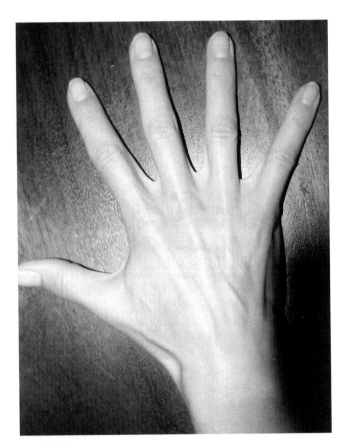

FIGURE 12-5

Finger fan = intrinsic function intact.

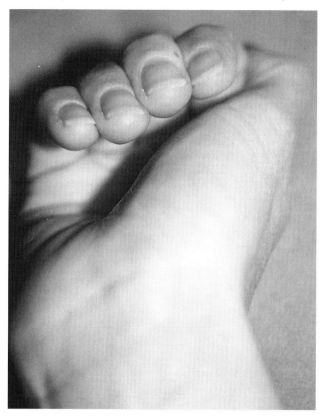

FIGURE 12-6

Normal cascade of fingernails with MP joints flexed. This checks for rotational deformity with metacarpal neck fractures compare the nail cascade to the uninjured hand.

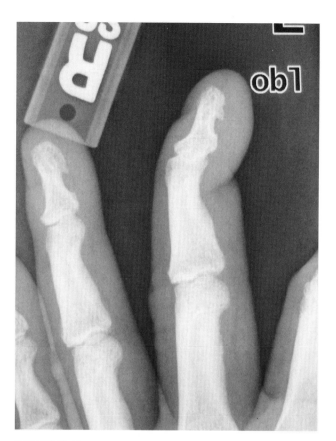

FIGURE 12-7

Mallet finger.

PROBLEM LIST

Mallet Finger (Fig. 12-7)

Patients may be unable to extend the DIP joint. There is a history of minor trauma with sudden loss of extension. A lateral view of the finger may show fracture of the dorsal part of the distal phalanx into the DIP joint. Splint these in full extension, even a bit of hyperextension. A paperclip wrapped in cotton and applied with narrow tape to the volar or dorsal side works well. Full extension at all times, without hurting the skin, is the goal. Instruct the patient not to let the joint bend, even a little and even for a second. Elevate, keep dry to avoid maceration, and follow-up within 5 days.

Jersey Finger (Fig. 12-8)

Patients present with a history of holding on by the fingertips as an opponent pulls away. The deep flexor rips away from the distal phalanx. Patients are unable to flex the DIP joint actively; passive flexion is fine. There may be a lump in the palm and a small fleck of

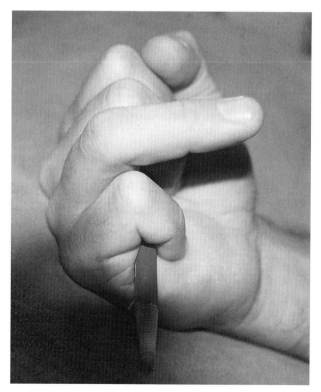

FIGURE 12-8

Jersey finger.

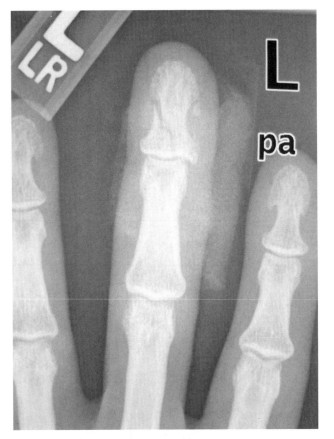
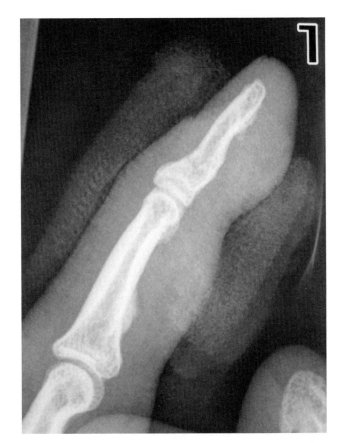

FIGURE 12-9

Open fingertip injury.

avulsed bone seen on the lateral film. The ring finger is the most common site.

Follow-up is most important. Early repair is the only chance of successful treatment. Splint with slight flexion of the wrist and MP and PIP joints to discourage the ripped tendon from retracting further up the hand. Make a next day appointment with the surgeon.

Open Fingertip Injuries (Fig. 12-9)

These involve some loss of tissue from the fingertip. Irrigate and debride meticulously. Spraying 1% plain lidocaine directly onto the open wound is a good way to start. Control the bleeding with gentle pressure—no tight wraps. Then call the surgeon (this is a plastic surgery referral in many hospitals). Although most of these injuries do fine with dressing changes alone, there are so many issues regarding the nail bed, cosmetic appearance, replantability of a severed tip, and the emotional trauma of loss and deformity that the person who ultimately is to be responsible for the patient's care should be involved from presentation. With a minor injury, you simply suture the laceration, give a

tetanus toxoid injection and an antibiotic, and send the patient home with 48-h follow-up instructions. Nevertheless, you should discuss this with the surgeon before sending the patient home.

DIP Joint Dislocation (Figs. 12-10 and 12-11)

These are often open injuries. Irrigate and debride, and then reduce the distal phalanx (which is almost always dorsally displaced) by pushing it with your thumb "off the end" of the middle phalanx. Do not pull on the finger tip. If you do this quickly and smoothly, it will hurt less than the anesthetic needle. Splint just the DIP joint in extension (i.e., leave the PIP joint free), and arrange for follow-up in 3 days or less. The reduction is quite stable.

Fractures of the Middle Phalanx (Fig. 12-12)

If displacement is less than 2 mm, you simply can apply an aluminum-foam splint and send the patient home with a 3-day follow-up. For greater displacement, you should attempt reduction by first getting

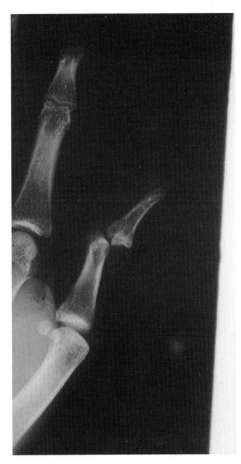

FIGURE 12-10

DIP joint dislocations.

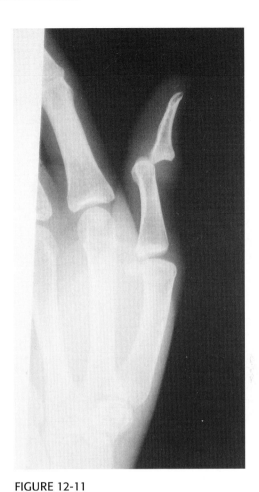

FIGURE 12-11

DIP joint dislocation.

angular alignment and then squeezing the fragments together. A splint can then be applied and the patient sent home, but follow-up should be within 24 h for displaced fractures because many are now treated with internal fixation. The splint should immobilize the DIP and PIP joints, but the MP joint is left free.

PIP Joint Dislocation (Fig. 12-13A and B)

This diagnosis may be made by history only; patients sometimes reduce this dislocation themselves when the notice "my finger went out of place." They will still have a good deal of swelling and tenderness around the PIP joint. If you have to perform the reduction, remember to *push* the middle phalanx off the end of the proximal phalanx using your thumb. Push it straight, don't pull it, because pulling can cause tissues to tighten around the base of the middle

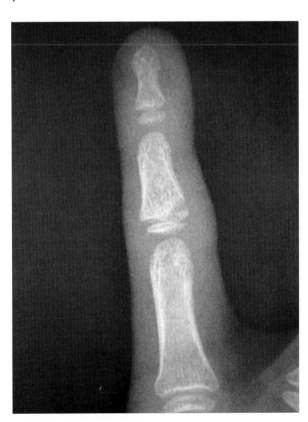

FIGURE 12-12

Fracture of middle phalanx. Salter II type.

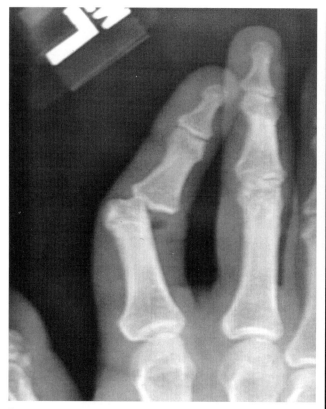

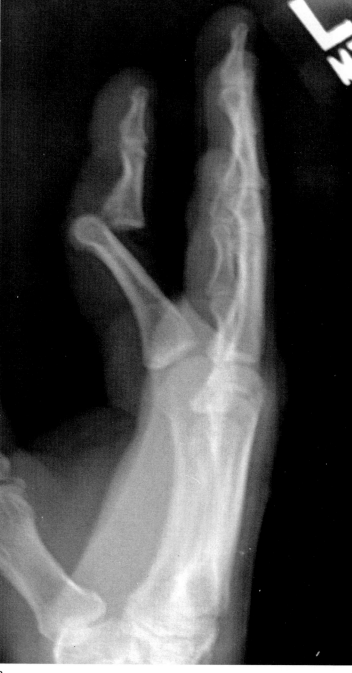

FIGURE 12-13

A. PIP joint dislocation. PA view *B.* PIP joint dislocation. Lateral view.   B

phlalanx, preventing the reduction. This is, nonetheless, a fairly easy reduction. Once reduced, this joint is fairly stable. Splint in extension, leaving the MP joint free, and schedule follow-up within 2 days.

Fractures of the Proximal Phalanx (Fig. 12-14)

If displacement is less than 3 mm, you simply can splint and arrange for 3-day follow-up. The splint

must immobilize the MP and PIP joints. Try to get the MP joint flexed to at least 40° and the PIP joint flexed less than 30°. If this position produces displacement of the fracture, however, it should be modified—fracture reduction comes first.

Displaced fractures should be reduced as well as possible and splinted, and the patient should be sent home with 24-h follow-up scheduled. The surgeon may want to internally fix these, and it is much easier within the first few days.

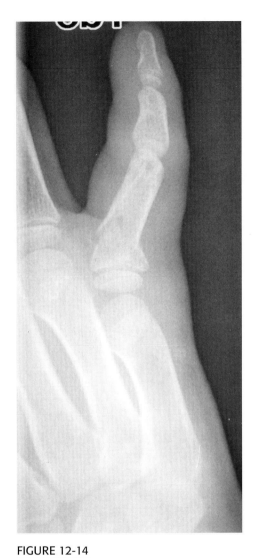

FIGURE 12-14

Fracture of proximal phalanx.

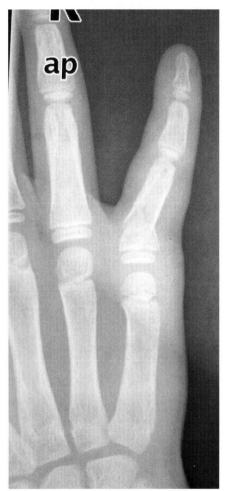

A

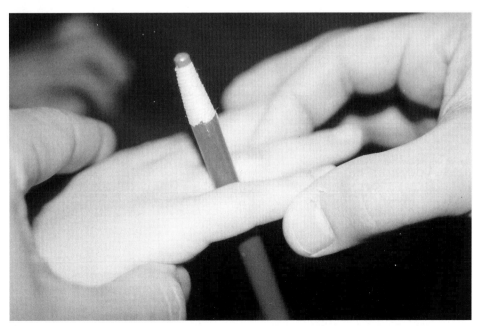

FIGURE 12-15

A. "Extra-octave" fracture at base of fifth proximal phalanx. *B.* Reductions maneuver for "Extra-octave" fracture.

B

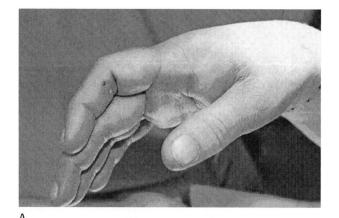

A

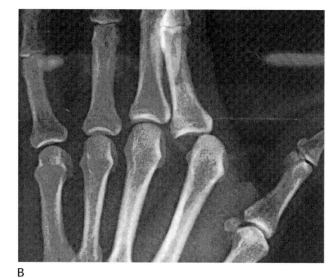

B

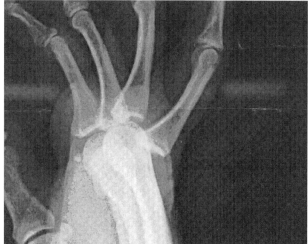

C

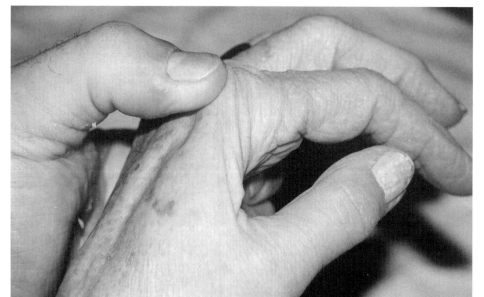

D

FIGURE 12-16

A. Clinical photo of MP joint dislocation. *B.* AP radiograph of index MP dislocation. *C.* Lateral radiograph of index MP dislocation. *D.* Reduction maneuver for index MP dislocation.

The "extra octave" fracture should have a good attempt at reduction in the emergency room where it is easiest. Reduce by putting a pen or pencil deep into the crotch of the web space and then squeezing the fourth finger to the fifth (Fig. 12-15A and B).

MP Joint Dislocation (Fig. 12-16)

Most often this is a dorsal dislocation. You always should attempt a reduction. Reduce by first extending the finger as far as possible (up to 90°) and then pushing the base of the proximal phalanx off the end of the metacarpal using your thumb—do not pull. Keep pushing until the MP joint reduces, and then flex it to 60°. Bear in mind that with pulling, the "Chinese finger trap" action of the tissues through which the proximal phalanx has gone tightens the rent, preventing the wider base of the phalanx from going back through and into its joint cavity. Even if done properly, a closed reduction may be impossible. This is termed a *complex dislocation*.

If you are able to reduce it, splint the MP joint loosely in slight flexion or "buddy tape" it to the next finger and send the patient home with 3-day follow-up instructions. If you cannot reduce it, call in the surgeon. He or she probably will make another unsuccessful attempt before bringing the patient to the operating room the next day.

Make sure to document the neurologic status of the involved finger because the dislocation stretches the neurovascular bundles.

Ulnar Collateral Ligament (UCL) Injury of Thumb

This is commonly called *gamekeeper's thumb*. The radiograph typically is normal, but look carefully for a small fragment of bone on the ulnar side of the thumb MP joint. The clinical sign of point tenderness at the UCL is a reliable sign of this injury (Fig. 12-17A). Laxity to applied valgus stress with the MP joint in about 30° of flexion is compared with the other side (Fig. 12-17B). Put the thumb in spica splint with the IP joint free (Fig. 12-17C).

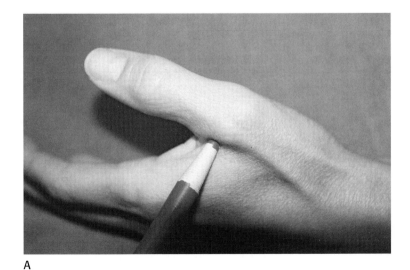

A

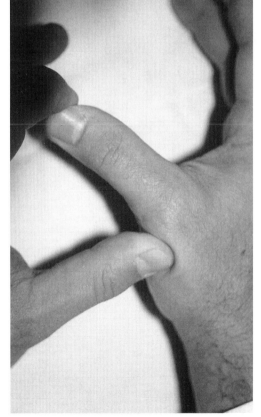

B

FIGURE 12-17

A. Ulnar collateral injury of thumb, tender spot. *B.* Valgus stress application.

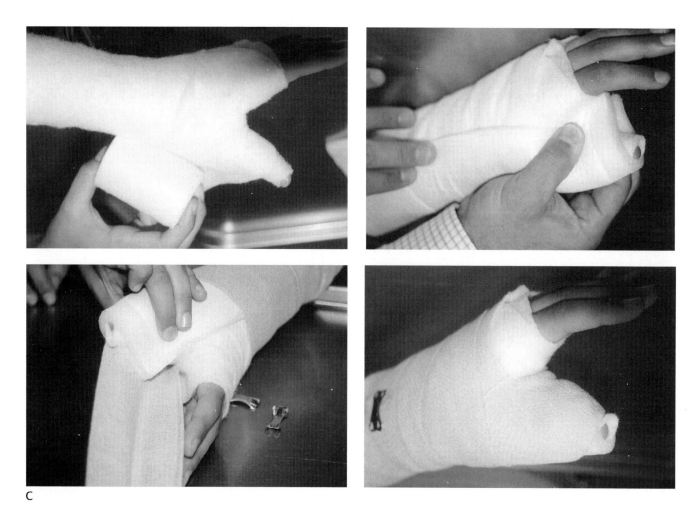

C

FIGURE 12-17

C. Thumb spica splint application.

13

Hand and Wrist: The Metacarpals and Carpals

NORMAL RADIOGRAPHS

Figure 13-1 shows posteroanterior (PA), lateral, and scaphoid views of hand illustrating the first metacarpal, trapezium, scaphoid, radial styloid, second metacarpal, trapezoid, third metacarpal, capitate, lunate, fourth and fifth metacarpals, hamate, triquetrum, pisiform, and ulnar styloid. You need to be able to accurately

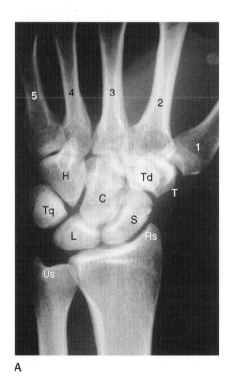

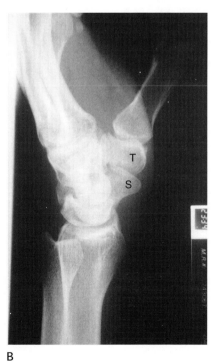

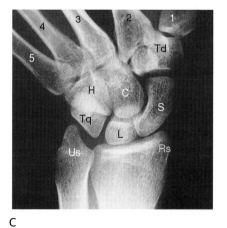

A

B

C

FIGURE 13-1

Normal hand. *A.* PA view. *B.* Lateral view. *C.* Scaphoid view. T = trapezium; S = scaphoid; Rs = radial styloid; Td = trapezoid; C = capitate; L = lunate; h = hamate; Tq = triquetrum; p = pisiform; U = ulnar styloid. (1) 1st metacarpal (2) 2nd metacarpal (3) 3rd metacarpal (4) 4th metacarpal (5) 5th metacarpal.

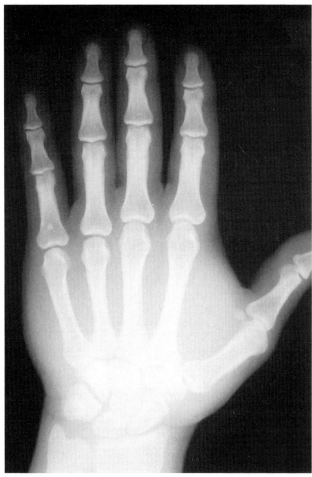

FIGURE 13-2

Soft tissue technique radiograph of hand. Note pronounced soft tissue swelling and location of MP joints with respect to web spaces.

FIGURE 13-3

A. Snuff box. (arrowhead) *B.* Dorsal and volar palpation of the scaphoid. *C.* Palpation of the radial styloid.

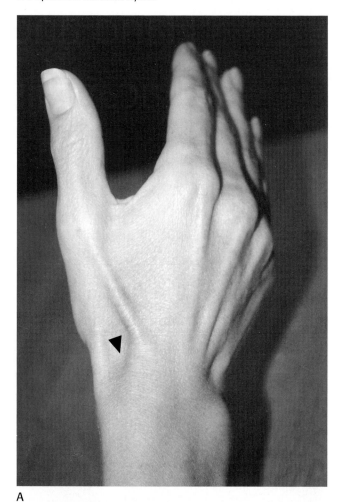

A

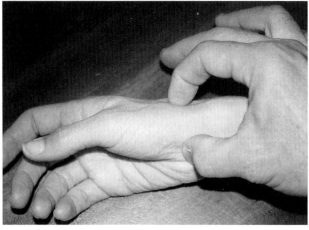

B

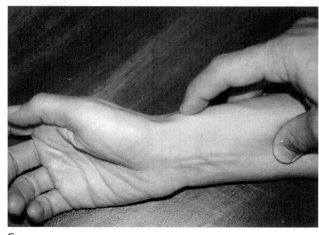

C

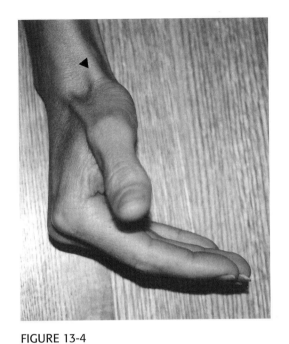

FIGURE 13-4

First dorsal compartment tendons (arrowhead).

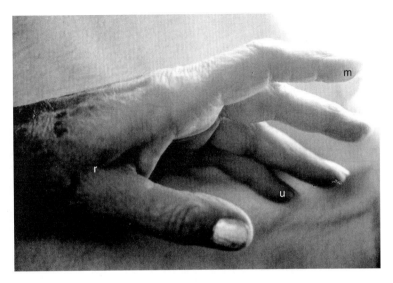

FIGURE 13-5

Median, ulnar, radial innervation zones. m = median; u = ulnar; r = radial.

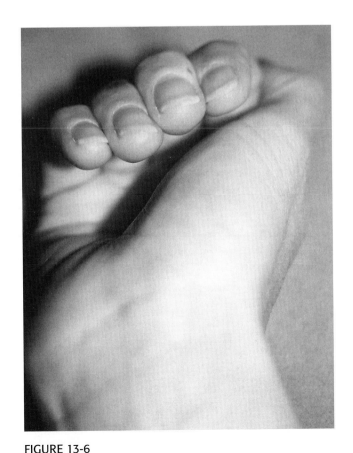

FIGURE 13-6

Cascade of fingernails.

palpate the scaphoid bone as tenderness here can indicate a fracture, even if radiographs are normal. The scaphoid can be palpated volarly, dorsally and radially in the anatomic snuff box. Be able to distinguish the scaphoid from the radial styloid. Figures 13-2 through 13-6 will help with this.

Fifth Metacarpal Fracture (Fig. 13-7A, B)

Metacarpal neck fractures are very common. Check the rotational deformity by flexing the MP and PIP joints while keeping the DIP joints extended; this is the most important problem to reduce. The cascade of the fingernails (see Fig. 13-6) should look the same as on the other hand. Reduce by pushing down on the dorsal side while holding the MP joint in flexion (Fig. 13-7C). Splint with thin plaster in an intrinsic plus position as in Fig. 13-7D. Check rotation again after reduction. These fractures often present when they are a few days old. Late reduction is more difficult. Orthopedic follow-up within 24 h will make sure that any additional reduction that you can achieve still will be relatively easy.

Metacarpal Shaft and Base Fractures (Fig. 13-8A, B)

Rotational deformity is very important to notice and reduce. Also look for dislocation or subluxation of the carpometacarpal (CMC) joint—this may be apparent

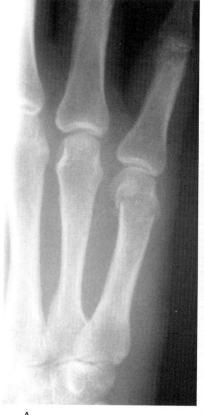

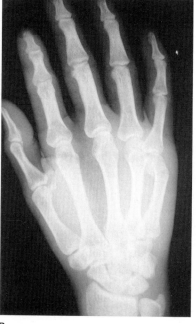

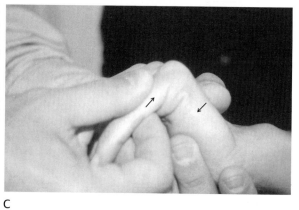

A   B   C

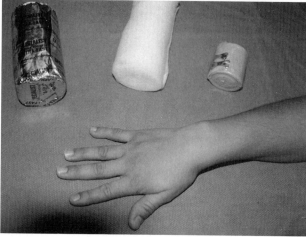

D-1 collect necessary materials: 4 inch plaster, cast-padding, elastic bandage.

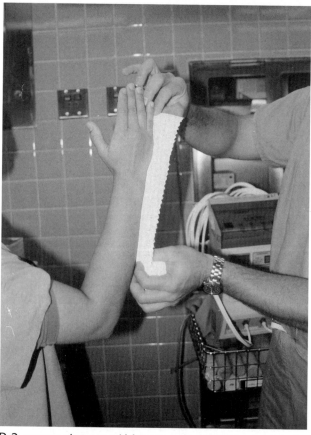

FIGURE 13-7

Fifth metacarpal neck (boxer's) fracture. *A.* Fifth metacarpal neck/head fracture – PA view. *B.* The classic "boxer's fracture." Lateral view. *C.* Reduction of boxer's fracture. Arrow shows direction of applied force. *D.* Splinting of boxer's fracture.

D-2 measure plaster to mid forearm make splint 6 layers of casting material thick.

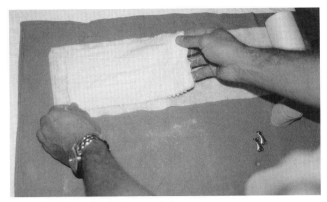

D-3 wet plaster. Express water and air.

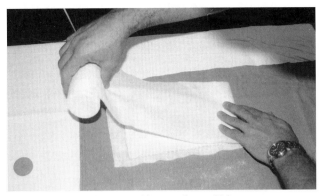

D-4 cover plaster with cast padding 1–2 layers thick.

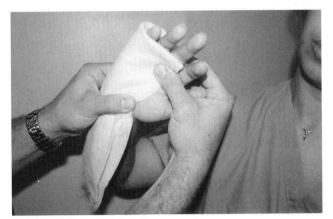

D-5 apply to ulnar hand forearm.

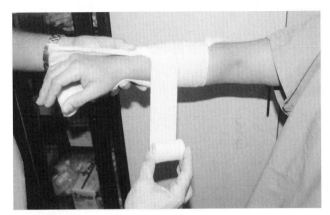

D-6 wrap on with elastic bandage.

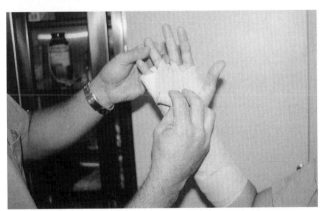

D-7 move quickly must reduce and mold before plaster sets.

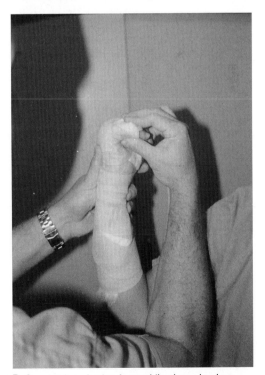

D-9 maintain reduction force while plaster hardens.

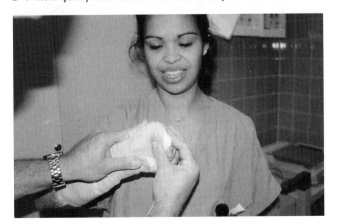

D-8 apply reduction.

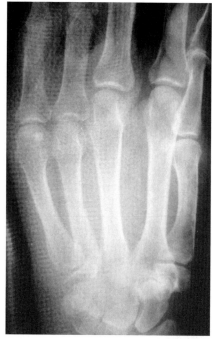

A

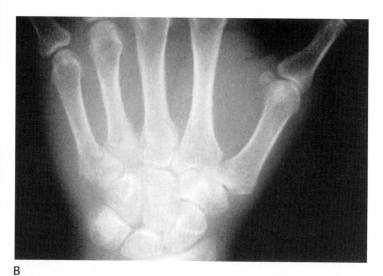

FIGURE 13-8

A. Metacarpal shaft fracture. *B.* Metacarpal base fracture. *C, D, E.* Ulnar gutter splinting.

B

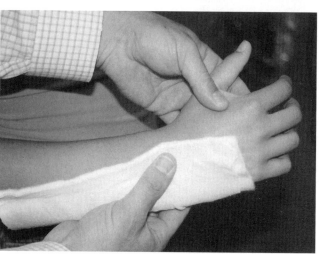

C

D

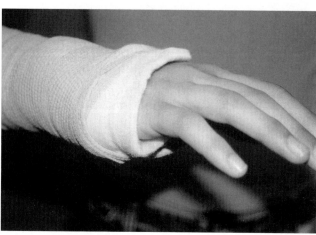

E

only on the lateral film. Thin padded real plaster of Paris splints should be placed volar and dorsal with the MP joint flexed and the IP joints extended allowing you to reduce the fracture within while they are hardening. Be careful to avoid "dents" while molding the plaster—these can produce skin damage, especially as the hand swells. See Fig. 13-8C, D, E for how to apply an ulnar gutter splint to 3rd, 4th and 5th metacarpal shaft and base fractures. Although patients with these injuries all can be splinted and sent home with 24-h follow-up instructions, it is good practice to call the surgeon on call because he or she may want to admit this patient for open reduction and internal fixation (ORIF); it is a judgment that he or she will make.

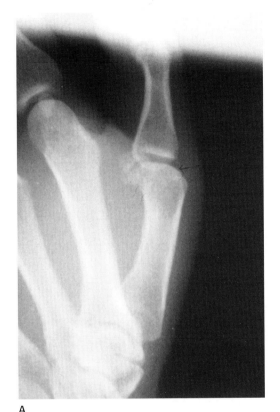

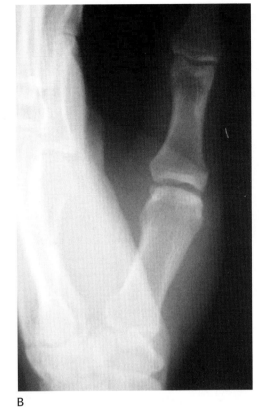

A   B

FIGURE 13-9 A,B

Fracture of first metacarpal head and neck.

The second, third, and fourth metacarpals are much less mobile than the first and fifth. Deformity from a poorly reduced fracture therefore is more difficult to tolerate. The degree of swelling that usually is seen with these injuries makes control of the bone by casts and splints quite difficult. It is therefore quite likely that a displaced or angulated fracture will need ORIF. So call the surgeon about all of these. If he or she does not want to operate acutely, you can put on a well-padded volar splint from the midforearm to the PIP joints and send the patient home with elevation and 36-h follow-up instructions. Remember to check the lateral film for CMC dislocation (see Fig. 13-12).

First Metacarpal Fractures (Fig. 13-9)

Fractures of the head and neck can be impaction-type with little swelling. They are easily missed. These fractures cannot be reduced easily, but they do well with a simple radial thumb spica splint. Midshaft fractures often are displaced. They can go into the same thumb spica splint, but put this on with cooler water and try to reduce the fracture with traction and direct pressure while the splint is hardening. Some surgeons do operate on these, so be sure to call the

surgeon about all displaced or angulated fractures. It is safe to send these patients home with 36-h follow-up instructions.

Fractures of the base of the first metacarpal usually displace due to the pull of the abductor pollicis longus. These are usually referred to as *Bennett's fractures* (Fig. 13-10*A*), although hand surgeons refer to those with comminution of the ulnar part of the metacarpal base as *Rolando's fractures*. Reduce by applying axial traction with your fingers while pushing the base of the metacarpal back where it came from with your thumb (Fig. 13-10*B*). Keep doing this while the padded radial thumb spica splint of 4-in. plaster (that you apply using cool water) is hardening. Many of these fractures require ORIF, so call the surgeon. The patient can go home with 24-h follow-up instructions if the surgeon does not want to admit the patient for surgery.

Carpometacarpal Dislocations and Fracture Dislocations (Figs. 13-11 and 13-12)

Sometimes obvious but often quite difficult to see, these injuries are obscured on examination because of the tremendous ability of the dorsal hand tissues to

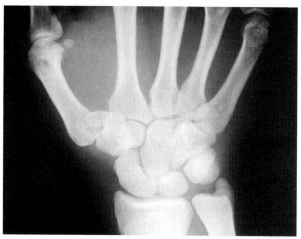

A

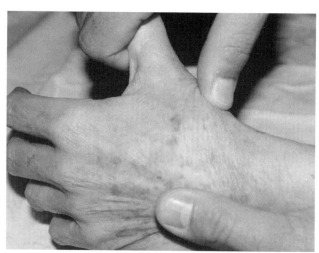

B

FIGURE 13-10

A. Fracture of first metacarpal base (Bennett's fracture).
B. Reduction maneuver for fracture of first metacarpal base.

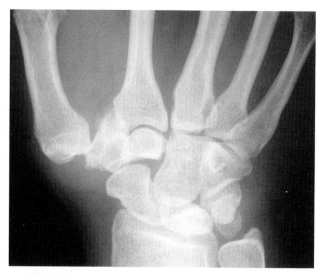

FIGURE 13-11

First Carpometacarpal dislocation.

swell. A good lateral x-ray is the best way to find these injuries. The patient will generally be able to show you where it hurts—it will be tender here—and the lateral film will show you the base of the metacarpal sticking up dorsally, if only by a small amount (Fig. 13-12). Do not miss a metacarpal fracture (often associated). Put on a volar splint up to the PIP joints with the MP joints flexed, and send the patient home with 36-h follow-up instructions. You may try to push the base back down. This is hard unless you apply a good deal of traction

and the patient relaxes. It also has a good chance of popping right back up when you release the pressure. This is why orthopedists pin many of these.

Scaphoid Fractures (Fig. 13-13)

The scaphoid or carpal navicular is shaped like a peanut. It is covered with articular cartilage over most of its surface, leaving a very small area in the midbody of the bone for vascularization. Because of this unfortunate anatomy, a fracture can separate a portion of the bone from its blood supply. If healing and neovascularization across the fracture site are delayed, the result can be avascular necrosis and a chronically painful, stiff, and arthritic wrist.

Scaphoid fractures are common. They are also commonly missed. Many nondisplaced scaphoid fractures are completely invisible on x-ray; the bone is broken, but the x-ray is truly normal. The *most* reliable sign of a scaphoid fracture is direct tenderness of the scaphoid-to-fingertip palpation. MRI is probably as sensitive as and more specific than your physical examination. Wrist MRI is not yet a must in the emergency room because you can treat the tender scaphoid as if it is fractured quite safely and cheaply. Simply put on a thumb spica splint, and send this patient home. In the emergency room, the scaphoid is considered fractured if it is tender.

Be very suspicious of a scaphoid fracture in any patient with wrist pain, especially radial side pain, after trauma. Get the plain films, and look at them carefully.

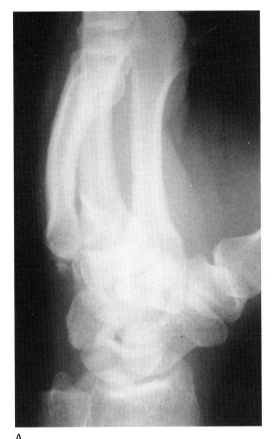

A

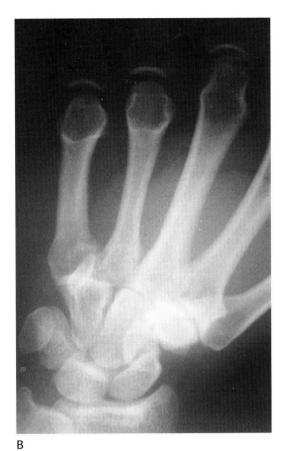

B

FIGURE 13-12

Carpometacarpal dislocation. *A.* Seen best on lateral view. *B.* Carpometacarpal dislocation–difficult to appreciate on AP view.

Special scaphoid views should be obtained if the pain is clearly around the scaphoid or if the scaphoid is tender. If the film shows a fracture *or* if the scaphoid is tender (even with the film normal), put the patient into a thumb spica splint (Fig. 13-13*E*) and a sling. This is quick and easy and can avert tremendous medical and legal problems. Call the orthopedist with your findings—especially when the fracture is displaced. He or she may want to admit the patient for ORIF or to put a cast on in the emergency room. Some use a long-arm cast, some a short-arm cast. This can be decided on later, though. The thumb spica splint with the arm in a sling is used most often in the emergency setting because it permits swelling better than a full-round cast. Nondisplaced fractures, once they have been put into the spica splint, can be followed up within 36 h.

Do not fail to take a look at the scaphoid when treating the very common distal radius fracture. Both can be fractured in the same injury, or the scaphoid may have a preexisting nonunion. Just make sure that the thumb ray is immobilized when you apply the splint for the radius.

Dorsal Avulsion Fractures (Fig. 13-14)

Pain with tenderness and swelling on the dorsal aspect of the wrist following trauma is the history given by patients with this fairly common problem. The PA film generally is normal. On the lateral views, however, it is clear that some bone has been separated from the dorsal aspect of the carpus. The origin of this bone is probably the lunate or triquetrum. It is often impossible to tell exactly which bone it is from. Treatment is the same for all of these. Apply a premade cock-up splint (or you can make your own padded volar splint of 3-in. plaster if necessary), and send the patient home with instructions for elevation, ice, and 72-h follow-up.

Trapezium Fractures (Fig. 13-15)

Direct local tenderness at the thumb CMC joint is the tipoff for trapezium fractures. An alert patient will show you exactly where it hurts. A question to ask the patient is whether it was painful there before the

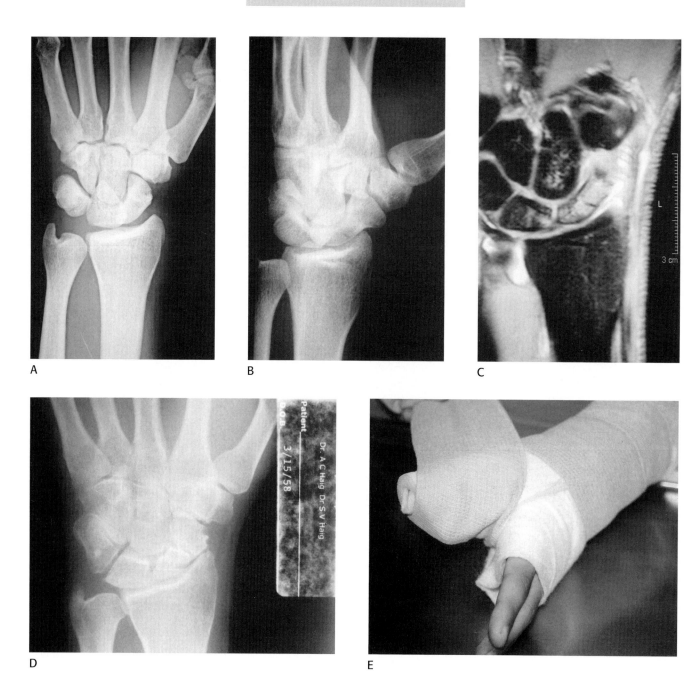

A   B   C

D   E

FIGURE 13-13

Scaphoid fracture. *A.* PA view normal *B.* Fracture visible on lateral and scaphoid views. *C.* Magnetic resonance imaging (MRI) confirms fracture. *D.* Old scaphoid fracture. *E.* Thumb spica splint (see also Fig. 13-12).

trauma. The trapezium is commonly encrusted with osteophytes produced by osteoarthritis of the joints it creates with the thumb metacarpal on its distal surface and the scaphoid on its proximal surface. Together these are called the *basal joint* of the thumb. Trauma to the thumb ray may crush or crack the bone, or it can break off some of the marginal flanges of oseophytes. In either case it is a fairly minor fracture that is well-treated with a thumb spica splint and 72-h follow-up.

Hamate Fractures

The hook (or hamulus) of this bone is the hard bump you palpate in the "heel of the hand" in line with the ulnar border of the ring finger. Direct trauma to this spot or more often holding onto a golf club, hammer, or baseball bat that hits something hard can result in a fracture of the hook of the hamate. It is a very hard fracture to see on plain films; even the special views

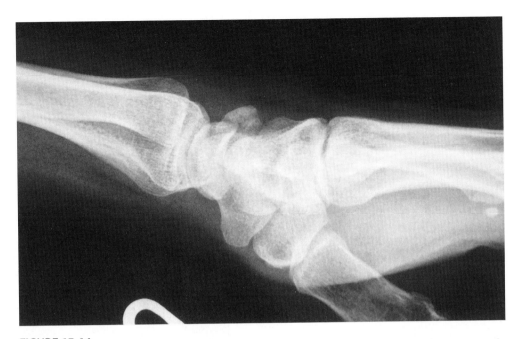

FIGURE 13-14

Dorsal carpal avulsion fracture.

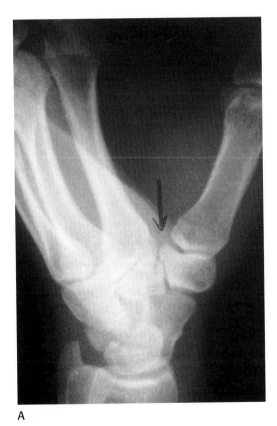

A

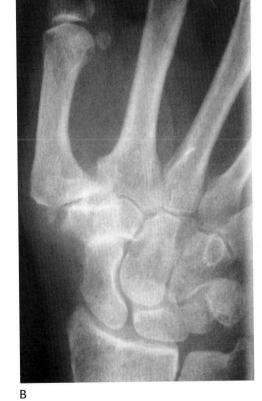

B

FIGURE 13-15

Fractures of trapezium. *A.* Without arthritis. *B.* In presence of paratrapezial arthritis.

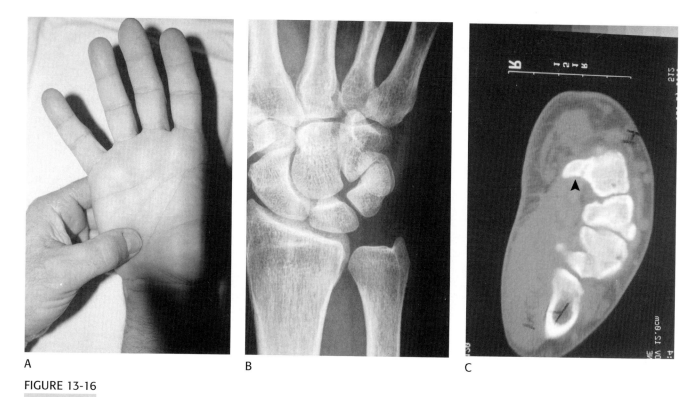

A   B   C

FIGURE 13-16

Fracture of hook of hamate. *A.* Tender spot in palm *B.* Plain film radiograph *C.* CT scan. Arrowhead shows fracture.

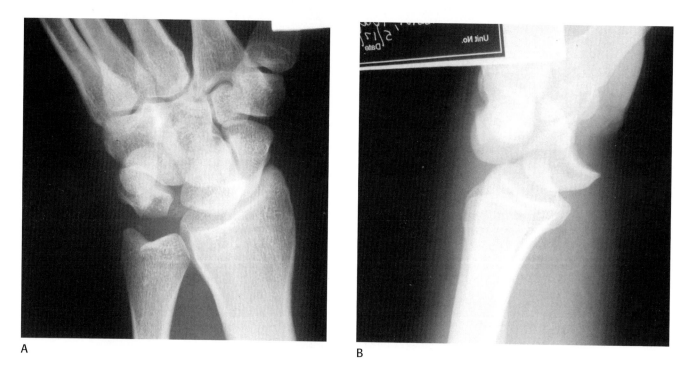

A   B

FIGURE 13-17

Perilunate dislocation of the carpus. *A.* AP view *B.* Lateral view – note empty lunate.

may not show it. Local tenderness of the hook is how the diagnosis is most often made (Fig. 13-16 *A, B, C*). The body of the hamate is fractured in direct hand trauma or crushing injuries.

Both of these injuries should receive a volar splint—the ready-made foam and Velcro type works fine. Follow-up should be within 48 h.

Capitate, Lunate, Trapezoid, Triquetrum, and Pisiform Fractures

All these little bones can be fractured by direct impact or some combination of twisting and crushing forces. As long as there is no major separation of the fragments and no dislocation of the corresponding joints, these are all safely treated with a volar splint, elevation, and 2-day follow-up. Make sure that there is definite tenderness where you think the fracture is. The lunate is the most common of these; the rest are uncommon.

Carpal Dislocations and Instability (see Fig.13-17)

A "sprained wrist" with normal motion, normal plain films, and pain at the end of the dorsiflexion or volar flexion range is a common emergency room diagnosis. This patient should get a wrist splint and 3-day follow-up instructions.

Dislocation of the carpus usually involves the capitate coming out of the concavity of the lunate (the "cup of the lunate"). This is best seen on the lateral radiograph. The PA film will be abnormal too; the wrist looks too short, and the joint spaces, which should all be pretty much the same, will seem too wide or too narrow. Check this patient for median nerve sensation—light touch on the volar aspect of the thumb, index, and long fingers. Call the surgeon and describe your findings. Emergency closed reduction and pinning often are necessary here.

Between wrist sprain and carpal dislocation there exists a wide spectrum of injuries to the soft tissues that hold the wrist together. Hand surgeons cannot yet agree on what to call these ligaments, let alone the specific injuries they sustain alone and in concert. When the x-ray is nearly normal—perhaps a bit of extra space between the scaphoid and lunate on PA view, the emergency physician should put the patient into a comfortable wrist splint and send him or her home with ice, elevation, and an appointment. When the x-ray is clearly abnormal—the lunate seems dislocated from the carpus or radius (Fig. 13-17), a joint space gap is half the width of a carpal bone, or there is an associated fracture of the scaphoid or radial styloid—you must call the orthopedist to evaluate. The specific diagnosis and treatment of the more subtle cases of traumatic intercarpal instability are also complex and controversial. The proper emergency treatment is clear, though—put the wrist in a splint.

14

Forearm and Elbow: The Radius and Ulna

NORMAL RADIOGRAPHS (FIG. 14-1)

PROBLEM LIST

- Distal radius fractures with and without fracture of the distal ulna
- Distal radioulnar joint and ulnocarpal joint injuries
- Radiocarpal dislocations
- Radial shaft fractures
- Ulnar shaft fractures
- Both bone fractures of the forearm
- Radial head fractures
- Olecranon fractures
- Nursemaid's elbow
- Elbow dislocation

Fractures of the Distal Radius and Ulna

These are very common. You must be able to describe this fracture to the orthopedist in some detail; simply telling him or her that you have a 30-year-old man with a distal radius fracture is of little help in making the necessary treatment decisions.

Describe the fracture by:

1. The direction in which the distal fragment is displaced (e.g., dorsal, volar, radial, ulnar) and the degree of displacement and angulation (e.g., 1 cm of radial displacement and 30° of dorsal angulation). Some fractures are impacted; this is a collapsing or telescoping of the bone into itself. This is common in older women with osteoporosis. When the lunate seems to have been driven into the radial joint surface, it is called a *die-punch fracture*.
2. The number of fragments there are (one, two, or many). This is the *degree of comminution*.
3. The joints into which the fracture lines extend (e.g., radiocarpal, radioulnar, or both). A fracture that does not break into any joint is termed *extraarticular*.
4. The presence or absence of an ulnar styloid fracture.
5. Other factors such as skin condition (open or closed), swelling, and neurovascular compromise (i.e., Is the hand cold and blue? Are the median innervated fingers numb?).

FIGURE 14-1

Normal radius and ulna. *A.* Anteroposterior (AP) view. *B.* Lateral view.
C, D. Posteroanterior (PA) and lateral
views showing normal osseous anatomy but gas in soft tissues (gas
gangrene). R = radius, U = ulna, Rh =
radial head

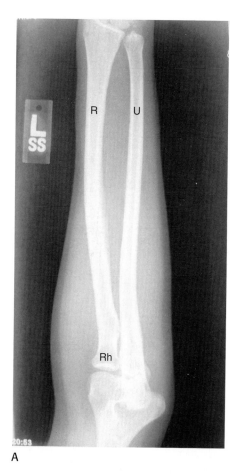

A

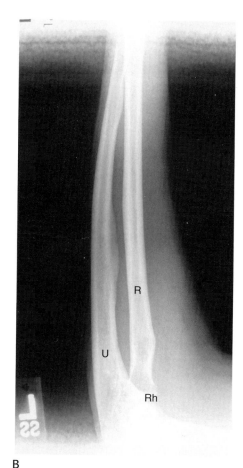

B

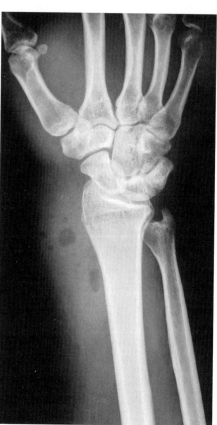

C

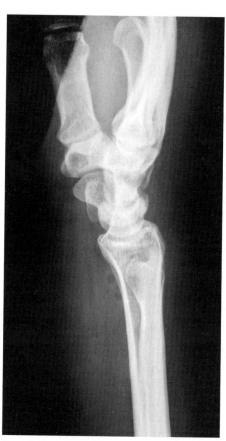

D

Common patterns to recognize include:

1. The dorsal lip fracture (usually called a *Barton's fracture*). This can permit dorsal subluxation of the entire carpus (Fig. 14-2).
2. Fracture of the volar lip is often called a *Smith's fracture* (Fig. 14-3), although *volar Barton's* is also used. As expected, this may permit volar subluxation of the entire carpus.

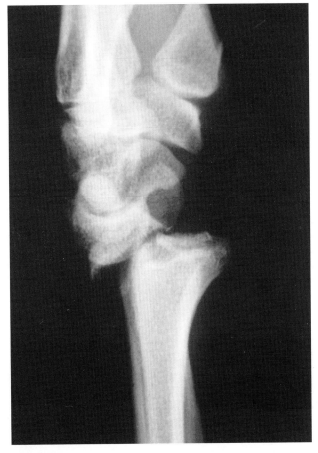

FIGURE 14-2

Dorsal lip fracture of the radius (Barton's). *A.* PA view. *B.* Lateral view.

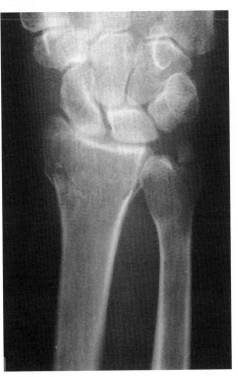

A

B

FIGURE 14-3

Volar lip fracture of the radius (Smith's). *A.* PA view. *B.* Lateral view.

3. A fracture that just knocks off the radial styloid is called a *chauffeur's fracture* (in early automobiles, the starter crank would spin when the engine caught, coming around to whack the poor chauffeur's radius) (Fig. 14-4).

4. The die-punch fracture in which the lunate is driven into the distal radial joint surface (Fig. 14-5). This plain film can be nearly normal, but the patient is definitely tender at the distal radius dorsally. On careful reinspection (even radiologists miss these), you may notice increased density of the bone just proximal to the joint surface. This is where the cancellous bone has been compressed or compacted.

5. The classic *Colles fracture* (Fig. 14-6) is displaced dorsally with dorsal and radial angulation, often somewhat impacted. *Colles* has been used loosely to indicate any fracture of the distal radius. You are best advised to abandon its use in favor of an anatomic description unless the wrist is so smashed that an anatomic description is difficult. *Really bad Colles fracture* in this case does get the idea across. Figure 14-6(*C,D*) shows an old, healed Colles fracture.

6. Children get torus or "buckle" fractures of the distal radius. The plain films show a wrinkling or buckling of the cortical bone (Fig. 14-7). They are essentially impacted and are quite stable.

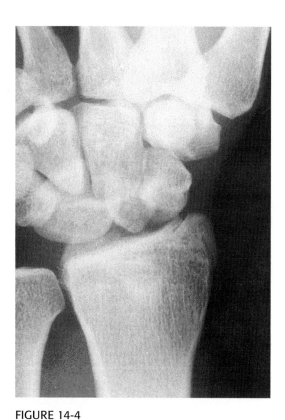

FIGURE 14-4

Fracture of the radial styloid.

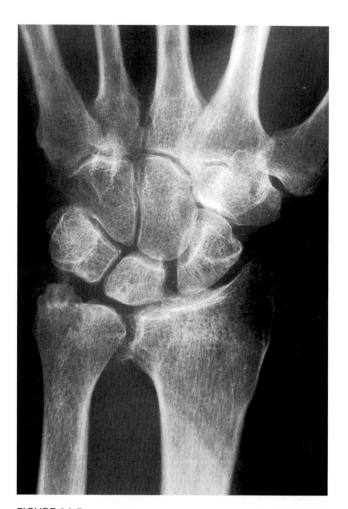

FIGURE 14-5

Fracture of the distal radius, lunate impaction or die-punch type.

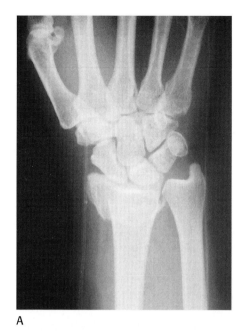

A

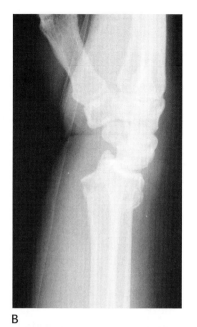

B

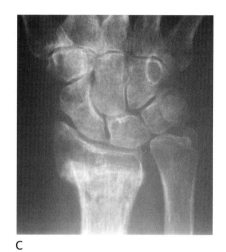

C

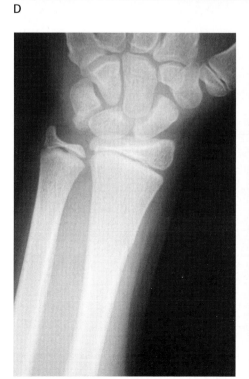

D

FIGURE 14-6

Fracture of the distal radius, typical Colles type. *A.* PA view. *B.* Lateral view. *C, D.* PA and lateral view of an old healed Colles fracture.

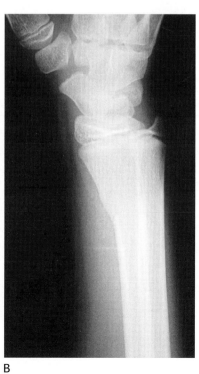

A   B

FIGURE 14-7

Fracture of radius, buckle or torus type. *A.* PA view. *B.* Lateral view.

TREATMENT

The ultimate goal with all these injuries is to reduce and immobilize them. In the emergency setting, the big question is, "Does someone have to come in right now to reduce this?" First, make sure that there is no neurologic or vascular compromise and that the little scrape on the skin is not actually a compounding wound (so probe it with a sterile cotton applicator stick). Then decide if immediate reduction is needed. With displacements smaller than 1 cm and angulations under 30°, a simple prefab splint, elevation, ice, Tylenol 3, and next day follow-up are usually adequate treatment for a distal radius fracture. Nevertheless, you should call the orthopedist before sending the patient home; the orthopedist may want to put a cast on the patient in the emergency room.

As the fracture gets uglier, the pain increases, the risk of neurovascular problems increases, the difficulty of getting an anatomic reduction increases, and the need for the orthopedist to come in *now* increases. This is why being able to accurately assess the fracture is so important.

Reduction of displaced distal radius fractures typically is performed by orthopedists and sometimes by their physician's assistants. This is a painful and rather difficult procedure in the emergency room. The experience that orthopedists have gained with these in the operating room, where there is an anesthetized patient and a fluoroscope, is what makes it easier for us in the emergency room. The basic maneuvers are shown in Fig. 14-8A. A volar splint (see Fig. 14-8B) is sufficient for fractures that did not require reduction. A sugar-tong splint generally is used if a reduction was performed (Fig. 14-9). Because these are commonly done in emergency rooms, you may gain facility through watching and being taken through some by orthopedists. The rule of thumb, however, is to call in the orthopedist for widely displaced fractures of the distal radius.

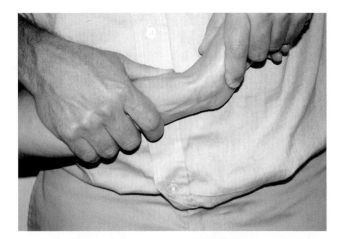

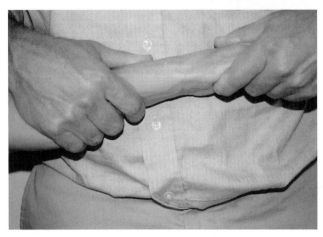

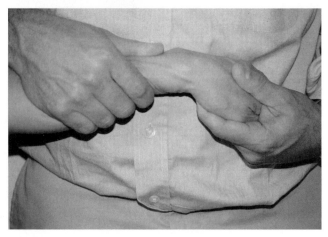

FIGURE 14-8A

Reduction of a Colles fracture.

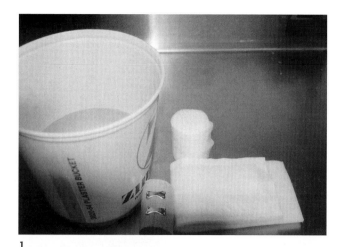

1

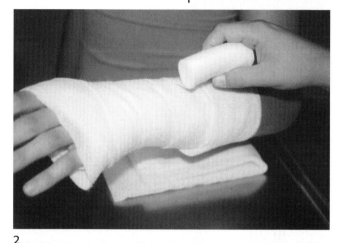

2

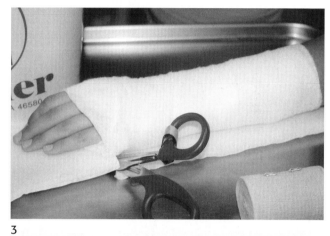

3

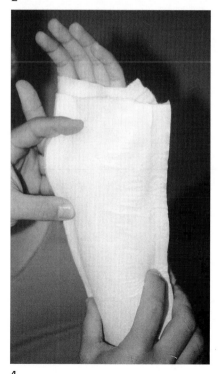

4

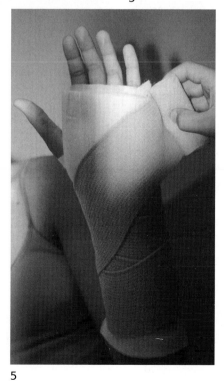

5

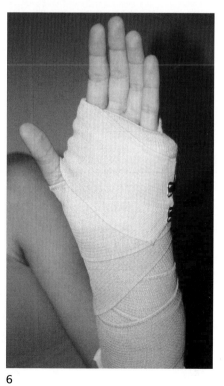

6

FIGURE 14-8B

Volar splint application.

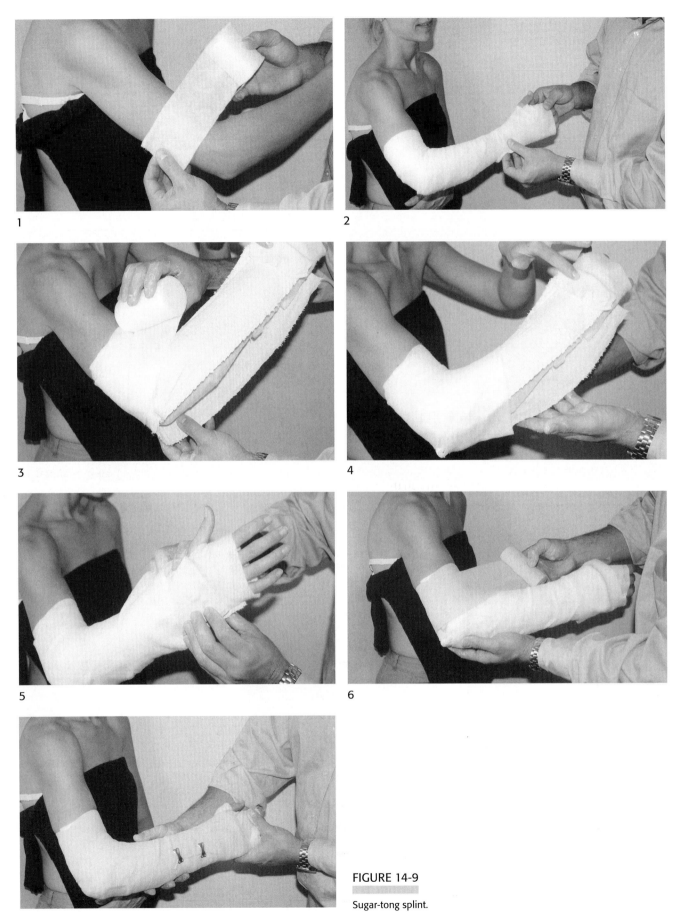

FIGURE 14-9

Sugar-tong splint.

Soft Tissue Injuries of the Radiocarpal, Ulnocarpal, and Distal Radioulnar Joint

A fall or a twisting injury produces most of these problems. The plain film shows no fracture. Swelling can be minimal to severe. With a radiocarpal sprain, the whole wrist is tender and swollen. This is a diagnosis of exclusion, though. Recheck the scaphoid. If it is the *most tender* spot, put on a thumb spica splint because you probably have a scaphoid fracture. Ulnocarpal and distal radioulnar joint sprains produce pain that is mostly on the ulnar side of the wrist. "Piano key" instability of the distal ulna is the most prominent sign of injury to the distal radioulnar joint. Tenderness in the interval between the ulnar styloid and the carpus is a sign of injury to the triangular fibrocartilage complex. This is the fibroelastic sheet that articulates with the ulnar part of the carpus and also holds the distal radius to the distal ulna. It is roughly a triangular hammock whose three supports are the ulnar styloid and the dorsal and volar corners of the ulnar side of the distal radius.

Put all these into a prefabricated cock-up splint, and send the patient home with instructions for elevation and 72-h follow-up.

Radial Shaft Fractures (Fig. 14-10)

There is commonly a fracture of the ulna or a dislocation of the distal radioulnar joint when the shaft of the radius is fractured. Look for these if they are not immediately apparent. All but minimally displaced, min-imally angulated (<1 cm, <10°) radial shaft fractures need to be seen by the orthopedist before the patient leaves the emergency room. Many require internal fixation. The minimally displaced fracture can be placed into a long-arm splint (Fig. 14-11) or a sugar-tong splint (see Fig. 14-9). Put the arm into a sling with ice, elevate overnight, and give the patient pain medication and instructions for 24-h follow-up.

Fracture of the radial shaft has been termed the *fracture of necessity*, meaning that it has to be treated surgically. Most of these are treated with a long plate held to the bone with screws. Getting the radial shaft back to its anatomic shape is the goal of this treatment; rotation of the forearm into pronation and supination is hindered if the shape of the radial shaft is not restored.

Rotational forces are to blame for most fractures of the radial shaft. These forces often injure the distal attachments of the radius to the ulna, i.e., the distal radioulnar joint. This combination, a radial shaft fracture (usually in the distal half) with a dislocation or subluxation of the distal radioulnar joint, is called a *Galleazzi fracture*. It needs internal fixation. The radiographic findings at the distal radioulnar joint may be subtle or nonexistent despite the soft tissues being badly injured. So whenever you see a fracture of the shaft of the radius, be sure to check for tenderness at the distal radioulnar joint. Check also along the entire shaft of the ulna (an ulnar shaft fracture is actually more likely to accompany the radial shaft fracture than a distal radioulnar joint injury). Splint this patient with a comfortable sugar-tong splint, and call the orthopedist to let him or her know that he or she has some work to do.

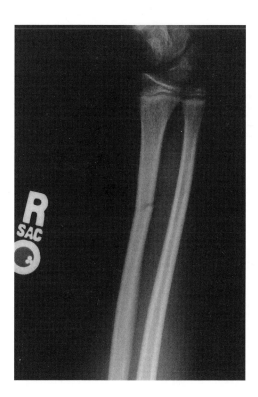
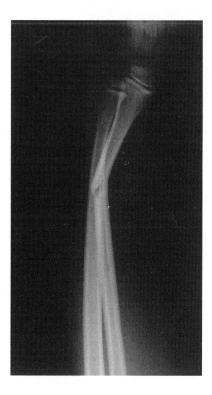

FIGURE 14-10

Radial shaft fracture.

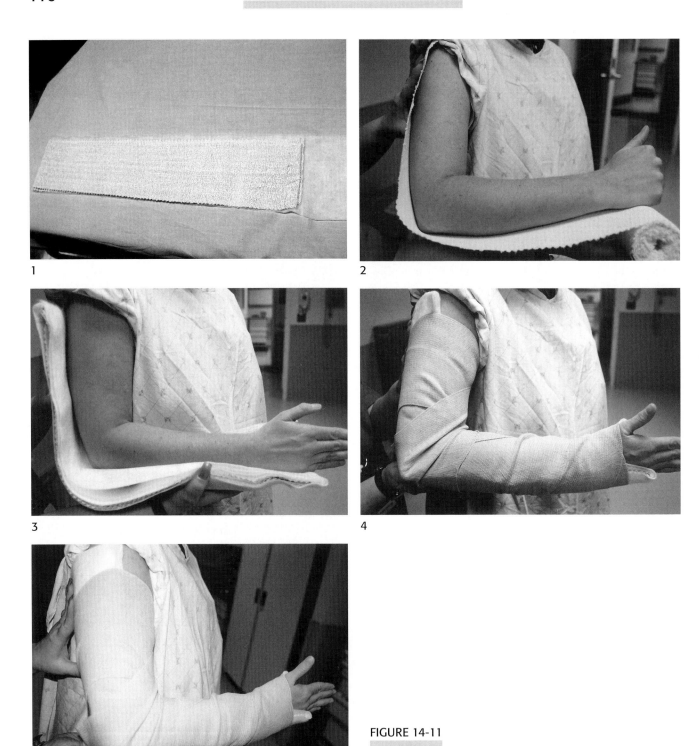

1

2

3

4

A

FIGURE 14-11

Long-arm splint.

Ulnar Shaft Fractures (Fig. 14-12)

Fractures of the shaft of the ulna are of two types. The *nightstick fracture* is produced by a direct blow to the subcutaneous shaft of the ulna. There is no other dislocation or fracture. The other type is called a *Monteggia fracture* (Fig. 14-13). This is a fracture of the ulna, usually the proximal half, with an accompanying dislocation of the radiocapitellar joint. It is produced most commonly by a fall that fixes the hand as the falling body rotates the forearm.

These mechanisms are sometimes reversed—a nightstick from a fall and a Monteggia from a direct blow. So take the history, but remember to examine the radiocapitellar joint. If it is tender or dislocated on x-ray, you have a Monteggia.

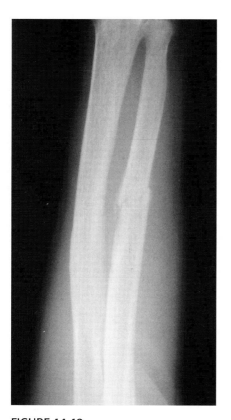
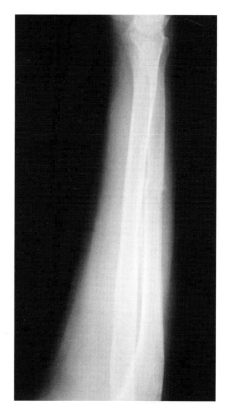

FIGURE 14-12

Ulnar shaft fracture.

These two are quite important to differentiate because the nightstick fracture can be put into a long-arm splint and the patient sent home with 48-h follow-up instructions, but the Monteggia fracture must be reduced and often fixed internally. The orthopedist must be called in for a Monteggia fracture; patients with this fracture are most often admitted for next day surgery.

The only Monteggia fracture for which the orthopedist does not have to come in is one in which the radial head and the ulnar fracture are completely reduced. In this case you will find tenderness but no radiographic dislocation at the radiocapitellar joint and a nondisplaced ulnar fracture. This patient can go home with a long-arm splint and instructions for 24-h follow-up.

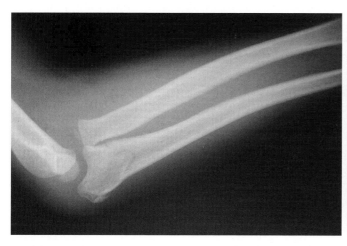
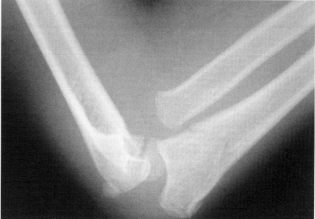

FIGURE 14-13

Ulnar shaft fracture with radiocapitellar dislocation—the Monteggia lesion.

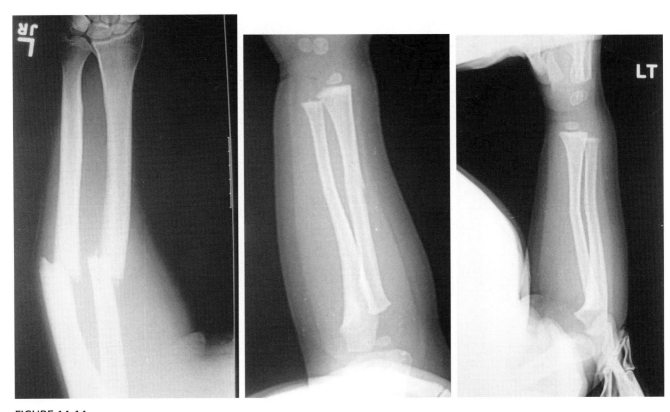

FIGURE 14-14

Fracture of radius and ulna shaft—the "both bones" fracture.

Fracture of Both Bones of the Forearm (Fig. 14-14)

The radius and ulna are both fractured proximal to the metaphyseal flare; i.e., the shafts of both bones are broken. This is a fairly common pattern, especially in children. If displacements are <1 cm and angulations are <15°, this patient can go home in a well-padded sugartong splint with instructions for 24-h follow-up—he or she probably will be treated with a cast. Do call the orthopedist, however, because he or she may want to reduce and cast the fracture in the emergency room. Also be sure to check the neurovascular examination on this patient and give instructions to elevate and monitor nerve function. Nerve laceration is rare, but forearm compartment syndromes are not.

Fractures of both bones with significant displacement or angulation are treated with open reduction and internal fixation (ORIF); most orthopedists use plates and screws for this. Admission for next day surgery is likely to be the orthopedist's choice for this patient. Call the orthopedist, and put the patient into a comfortable volar or sugar-tong splint (see Figs. 14-9 and 14-11 for how to make and apply these). Remember to make

plain films of the humerus and wrist/hand to check for concomitant fractures.

Radial Head Fractures (Fig. 14-15 and 14-16)

These are very common fractures. There is often no visibly broken bone on the plain films, only a "fat pad sign" (see Fig. 14-16) seen on the lateral view with reproducible tenderness at the radial head. The fat pad sign is caused by blood in the joint displacing anteriorly and posteriorly the fat pads that normally are right up against the distal humerus. They are dark triangles, like sails, anterior and posterior to the distal humerus. A tender radial head in the presence of a fat pad sign makes the diagnosis of radial head fracture. Remember that the olecranon tip, radial head, and lateral epicondyle of the humerus form a roughly equilateral triangle and that the radial head is easiest to palpate with the elbow in extension as you pronate and supinate the forearm. (Palpate your own before treating the patient.) This triangle is demonstrated in Fig. 14-17.

The fractures you diagnose this way are obviously nondisplaced. Many radial head fractures are displaced and therefore visible on the plain film. They are

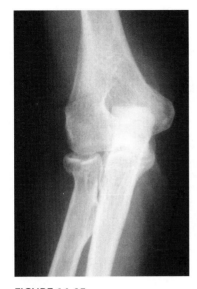
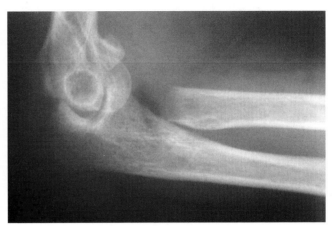

FIGURE 14-15

Radial head fractures.

seen most readily on lateral films of the elbow. Adults tend to fracture the head of the radius, whereas children more often fracture the neck of the radius.

The proper treatment for the vast majority of radial head fractures is completely counterintuitive. Do not wrap them up with Ace bandages. Do not splint them. You may give the patient a sling for comfort, but you should encourage him or her to remove it as soon as he or she can. The best treatment is to give the patient ice,

pain medicine, and a sling and tell him or her to move the elbow, without pressure or force, as much as he or she can. Follow-up with an orthopedist within 48 h is generally adequate.

Excellent studies have shown that the more these fractures are immobilized, the longer the elbow stays stiff. The orthopedist who follows up with this patient will need to make a decision about whether or not to operate on the elbow. The surgery usually consists simply of removing the entire radial head, although there are now some advocates of immediate prosthetic replacement or open reduction and fixation with special screws (remember that the entire surface is covered with articular cartilage). The decision to operate hinges largely on how well the patient regains elbow motion, and this is largely a function of how long the elbow is immobilized—although it is *also* related to the degree of displacement of the fracture fragments. So be sure to tell the patient that this is an unusual fracture that is best not immobilized.

Aspiration of the radiocapitellar joint with an 18-gauge needle often is suggested as a way to relieve the pain of this fracture, which can be considerable. The procedure is easy—just prep the skin with alcohol and Betadine, and aspirate slowly with a 10-ml syringe after putting the needle into the joint. It is right in the middle of the equilateral triangle formed by the olecranon, lateral epicondyle, and radial head. You should only be doing this if the joint is bulging with blood, making it easier to get your needle in. The decision to do an aspiration is based entirely on your

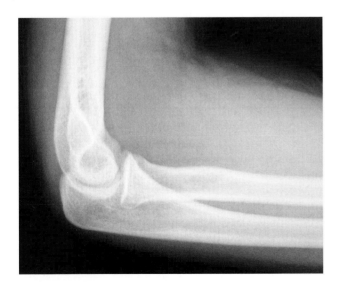

FIGURE 14-16

Fat pad sign on lateral film of the elbow.

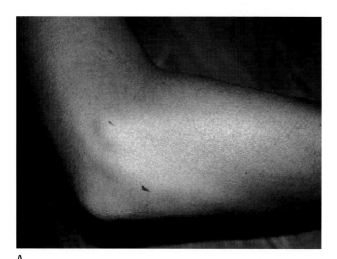

A

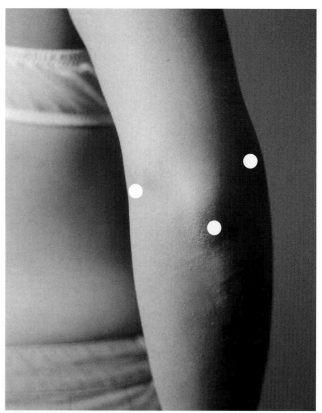

B

FIGURE 14-17

A. The lateral triangle of the elbow. *B.* The posterior triangle of the elbow.

judgment as to whether this patient's pain is that of the fracture and surrounding soft tissue injury, which aspiration will not help, or that of the tense hemarthrosis—blood under pressure in the joint—which will be relieved by aspiration. Most patients are scared to death of the needle anyway and will not let you perform the aspiration, especially after you have told them about your bizarre plan to use no cast and encourage early motion. Despite poor patient acceptance, aspirating just 2 ml from an acutely painful joint can make a very happy patient.

Olecranon Fractures of the Ulna (Fig. 14-18*A, B*) and Coronoid Process Fractures of the Ulna (Fig. 14-18C)

These are often avulsion fractures; the powerful triceps muscle, mighty extender of the elbow, can tear its own tendon, or more commonly, it tears apart the bone to which it is attached—the olecranon. Bearing in mind that the olecranon's anterior surface is the articulation of the ulna with the humerus, it should not be a surprise that just about all these fractures need to be fixed internally. Put the patient in a long-arm splint (see Fig. 14-11) , check the function of the ulnar nerve (which is quite nearby), and call the orthopedist for specific instructions. Many of these patients are admitted for next day surgery, although a high-functioning patient can be scheduled for surgery as an outpatient after office follow-up.

Much less commonly, the coronoid process, to which the brachialis muscle attaches, is avulsed by resisted elbow flexion force. Difficult but often necessary to repair, this fracture can be put into a long-arm splint and sling with 24-h follow-up, but the orthopedist must be alerted while the patient is still in the emergency room.

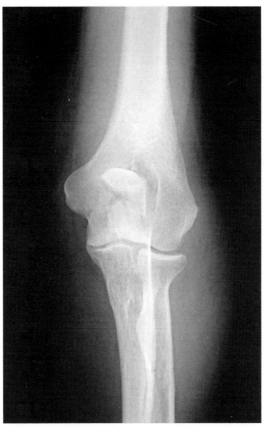

A Fracture of olecranon (AP view).

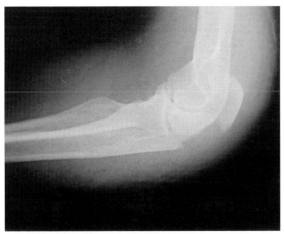

B Fracture of olecranon (Lateral view).

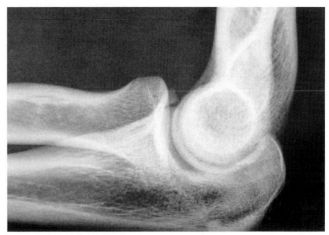

C Fracture of coronoid process (Lateral view).

FIGURE 14-18

Olecranon fracture. *A.* AP view. *B.* Lateral view. *C.* Coronoid process fracture.

Nursemaid's Elbow (Fig. 14-19)

A tearful child, old enough to walk but not usually old enough to talk, is brought in by his or her parent/caregiver, who looks sheepish. Someone big was holding the child by the hand and yanked—after which began the tears and refusal to use the arm at all.

On examination, there is obvious refusal to use the hand of the affected upper extremity; try holding out a dollar bill—most children will go for it with the unaffected hand. The neurovascular status seems normal. There is some tenderness to palpation of the lateral portion of the elbow anteriorly, but most children are screaming bloody murder whenever you put your fingers there. Obtain plain films of both elbows. They should be normal. Any type of fracture or abnormal relationship of the ossification centers on x-ray means that you are not dealing with a nursemaid's elbow.

The pathophysiology of this problem is that the annular or orbicular ligament, which surrounds the radial head, has slipped proximally off the radial head and into the joint. It is not all the way off, just partway

off. The adult who yanked the child's arm pulled the radius partway out of the ring.

The treatment for this problem is to supinate the child's hand (palm toward ceiling), put your thumb on the anterolateral forearm over the radial head (just distal to the elbow flexion crease), and then press down slightly with your thumb while flexing the elbow as far as it will go (Fig. 14-19). Try this a few times. A slight click may be felt as the radial head goes back into the annular ligament. You may feel nothing. Most of the time, however, the child suddenly seems fine and goes back to moving the elbow as if nothing happened. If it doesn't seem to work, try this maneuver a few more times. If there is still no improvement, call the orthopedist and describe the situation. He or she may want to make an attempt at the reduction, although many of these have been seen to be reduced when put into a sling overnight.

The reduced and happy nursemaid's child should be given orthopedic follow-up within 3 to 4 days. The patient does not need a sling, and if the examination is normal after you perform the reduction, the patient does not need a postreduction film (the prereduction film was normal).

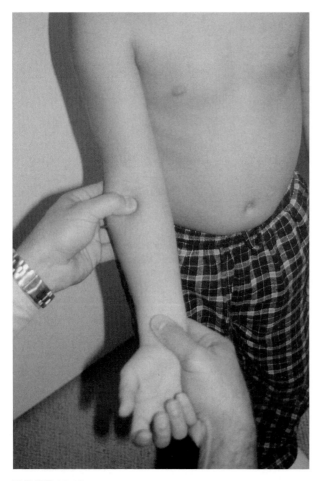 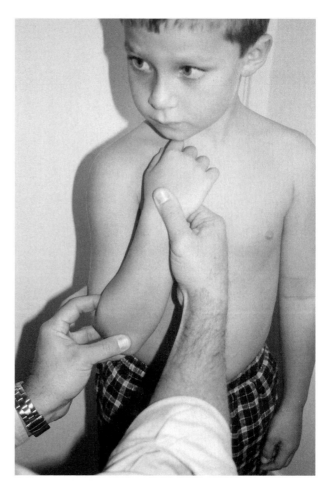

FIGURE 14-19

Reduction of nursemaid's elbow.

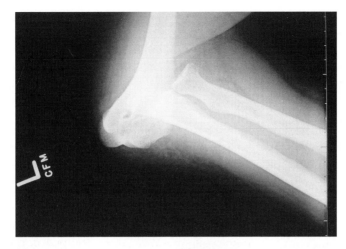

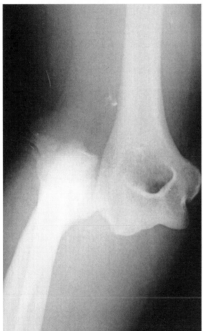
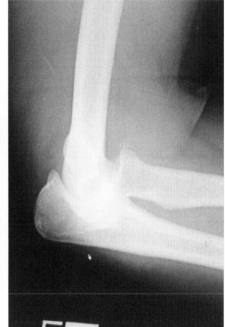

FIGURE 14-20

Elbow dislocation.

Elbow Dislocation (Figs. 14-20 and 14-21)

This patient has had a good bit of trauma—a fall or a fight. Tremendous pain accompanies this injury, and there is often numbness or weakness in the median or ulnar distribution. Plain films show that the humeral trochlea is not sitting in the semilunar notch of the ulna; the radial head may not be near the capitellum either, but it is the ulnohumeral relationship that is of primary concern. Most of the time the olecranon has gone posterior to the humerus. There is often an accompanying fracture of the medial epicondyle of the

humerus (this small piece sometimes lodges in the joint space, preventing proper reduction). Clinically confirm the dislocation by noting loss of the posterior triangle that normally is a nearly equilateral triangle formed by the olecranon tip and medial and lateral epicondyles (see Fig. 14-17B).

Make sure to record the neurovascular examination and give this patient pain medication. Then call the orthopedist. This is not a very difficult reduction to perform—it is actually easier than a shoulder—but it is far less common. The favored method of reduction is to apply a distal translocating force to the entire forearm

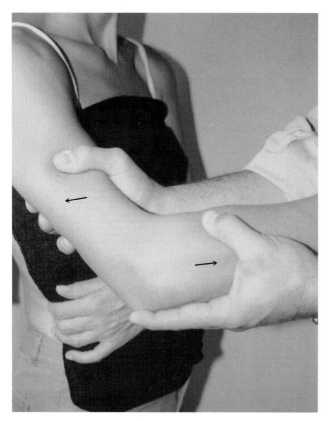

FIGURE 14-21

Reducing an elbow dislocation. Arrows indicate direction of applied force.

while pushing the olecranon anteriorly back under the humerus (Fig. 14-21). It is important that this be done gently. Let the orthopedist do this while you watch the first few times. There is no magic, but you need to know how hard to push. This is a much gentler reduction than the shoulder. After reduction, recheck and record the neurovascular examination, and apply a long-arm splint (see Fig. 14-11). Suprisingly, the bigger danger is overly long immobilization after closed reduction—we usually take them out and permit motion at a week.

If the elbow cannot be reduced in the emergency room, the patient must be taken to the operating room for reduction under anesthesia. There is often a fracture fragment blocking reduction. The median nerve also can be trapped in the joint—be sure to check its function.

Remember to order a sling, ice, oral pain medication, and follow-up within 48 h for the patient after reduction has been confirmed on postreduction plain films.

C H A P T E R

15

Humerus: Distal Humerus and Humeral Shaft

NORMAL RADIOGRAPHS

Figure 15-1*A, B* shows the distal humerus (elbow) with medial epicondyle, trochlea, capitellum, lateral epicondyle, olecranon fossa, transepicondylar axis, and capitellar axis. Note the normal anterior fat pad, humeral shaft, and ulnar groove. Figure 15-1*C* shows an elbow with no fracture but with osteoarthritis present. Figures 15-2 through 15-4 provide pediatric elbow films.

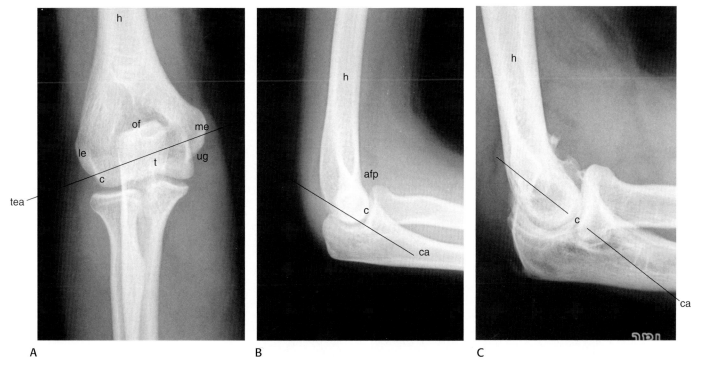

A   B   C

FIGURE 15-1

Normal distal humerus. *A.* Anteroposterior (AP) view. *B.* Lateral view. *C.* Arthritic elbow. me = medial eipcondyle; t = trochlea; c = capitellum; le = lateral epicondyle; of = olecranon fossa; tea = trans epicondylar axis; ca = capitellar axis; afp = anterior fat pad; h = humeral shaft; ug = ulnar groove.

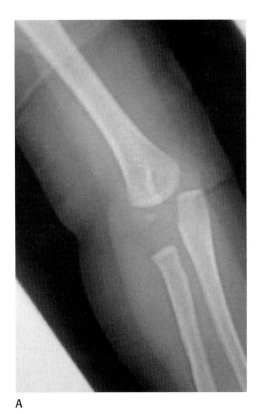

A

B

FIGURE 15-2

Elbow of a 1-year-old child. *A.* AP view. *B.* Lateral view.

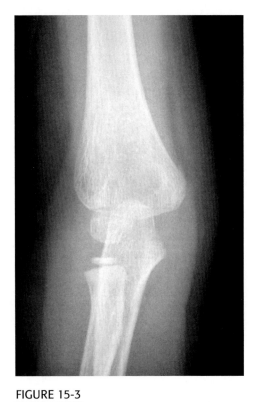

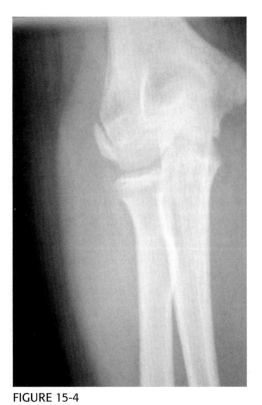

FIGURE 15-3

Elbow of a 5-year-old child. AP view.

FIGURE 15-4

Elbow of a 10-year-old child. AP view.

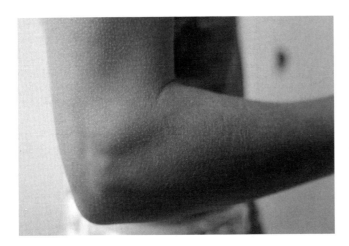

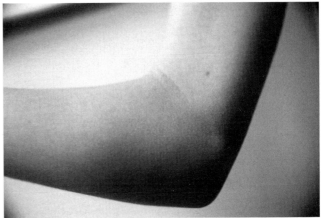

FIGURE 15-5

Elbow surface anatomy.

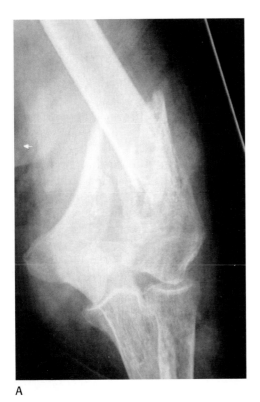

A

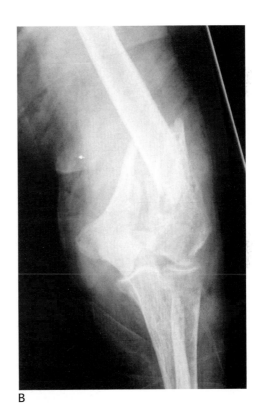

B

FIGURE 15-6

Supracondylar fracture. *A.* AP view. *B.* Lateral view.

ANATOMY (FIG. 15-5)

PROBLEM LIST

Supracondylar Fractures (Fig. 15-6)

These are above the joint surfaces but below the shaft. Generally they are caused by a fall onto the out-stretched hand. The patient has elbow pain and swelling and does not permit movement of the elbow, which is tender at or above the epicondyles.

If this fracture is displaced, the radiographs are obvious—showing a fracture above the transepicondylar axis (not actually into the joint but in the distal flare of the humerus). The distal portion usually is displaced and angulated posteriorly. There also may be medial or lateral angulation, displacement, or even rotation. The

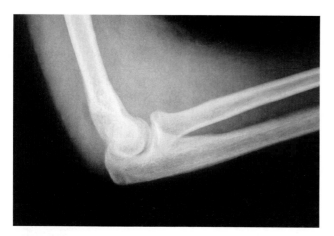

FIGURE 15-7

Posterior fat pad sign on lateral film of elbow.

radial head is still in normal contact with the capitellum, however, and the olecranon is normally related to the trochlea of the humerus.

These fractures are often nondisplaced. In this case, look for anterior and posterior fat pad signs—black triangular sails flown fore and aft from the distal humeral shaft on the lateral film (Fig. 15-7). This is caused by blood in the joint. Look at the lateral view; check for a subtle fracture line in the anterior or posterior cortex (Fig. 15-8). Also check the lateral view carefully for straightening of the capitellar axis angle (Fig. 15-9). This is a line drawn right down the middle of the capitellum. It should make an angle of about 135° with the line of the humeral shaft. It is always a good idea to get a film of the other elbow for comparison, even in an adult, if you have any doubt about a suspicious line or angle. Patients usually like this too.

Most supracondylar fractures are of the extension type (Fig. 15-10). This means that the elbow is hyperextended, breaking the humerus just above the joint and taking the distal, broken-off portion posteriorly into extension. The angle made by the capitellar axis and the humeral shaft therefore will be increased, making the capitellar axis more parallel to the humeral shaft. Check for specific localization of tenderness—this is the most reliable sign of a subtle fracture.

A displaced supracondylar fracture is obvious on the plain films. Remember that the fracture lines with a supracondylar fracture stay above the joint surfaces; the articular segment is all one big, intact piece. It may not be clearcut as to whether no fracture line actually goes into the condylar area. There is often quibbling about whether a fracture is supracondylar, intercondylar, transcondylar, epicondylar, or simply condylar. In the emergency room, the most important categories are simply displaced or nondisplaced because the nondisplaced fractures can be safely put into a long-arm splint and the patient sent home with 48-h follow-up instructions, whereas patients with displaced fractures need to be admitted for reduction, usually with internal fixation.

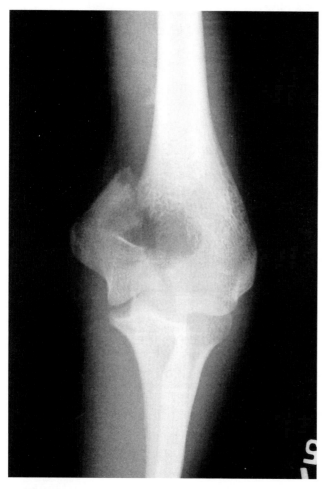

FIGURE 15-8

Condylar fracture.

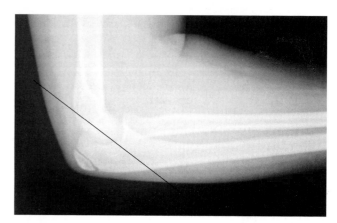

FIGURE 15-9

Capitellar axis drawn on lateral view of elbow.

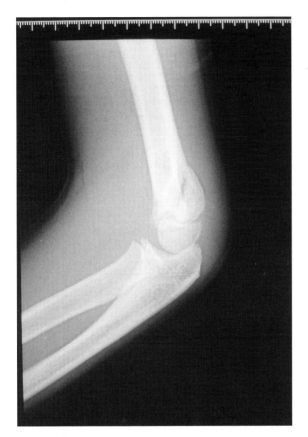

FIGURE 15-10

Supracondylar fracture, extension type—lateral view.
Note straightening of the capitellar axis.

TREATMENT

Supracondylar Fracture of the Humerus

Check and record ulnar, median, and radial nerve function. Immobilize all these nerves with a long-arm splint (see Fig. 14-11). Call orthopedics. A patient with a neurologically intact, nondisplaced fracture can go home with the splint, a sling, ice, pain medicine, and instructions for 48-h follow-up. A displaced fracture needs reduction under anesthesia and, often, internal fixation. Plenty of nerve injuries accompany these fractures, so be sure to look for them.

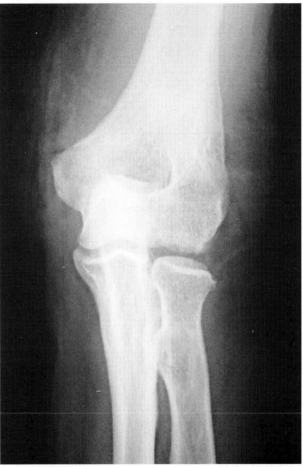

A

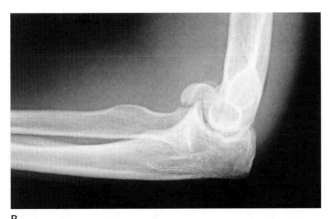

B

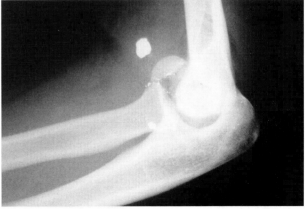

C

FIGURE 15-11

Capitellar fractures. *A.* AP view. *B.* Lateral view. *C.* Lateral view with bullet.

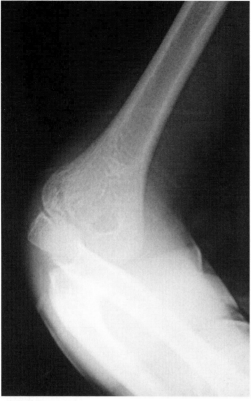

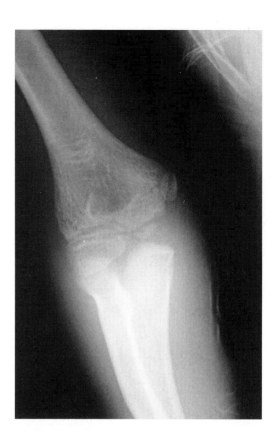

FIGURE 15-12

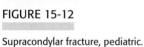

Supracondylar fracture, pediatric.

With the possible exception of medial epicondylar fractures, displaced distal humerus fractures are quite serious and difficult to treat. Up to a third of patients, despite optimal treatment, end up with permanent loss of motion. Keep this in mind when treating these patients. A positive impression of your care and concern is essential.

Intercondylar, Transcondylar, Condylar, Trochlear, and Capitellar Fractures (Figs. 15-11 and 15-12)

There are many anatomic variations, but all are fractures below the transepicondylar axis. Try to identify the major fracture lines, noting degree of displacement and how much comminution there is. Your call to the orthopedist must stress that there is a fracture of the distal humerus that goes into the joint, what portions of the joint are involved, and how displaced and comminuted it is. A patient with a truly nondisplaced fracture can go home in a long-arm splint with 24-h follow-up. Always call the orthopedist. Always document distal neurologic examinations. These are all difficult and dangerous fractures. Most require surgical fixation. Many patients do poorly even with optimal treatment.

Medial and Lateral Epicondylar Fractures

The medial epicondyle is avulsed in children, and it is knocked off the humerus by a direct blow in adults. It is a common fracture (Fig. 15-13). The lateral epicondyle fracture, on the other hand, is quite unusual. What you think is a lateral epicondylar is probably a lateral condylar or capitellar fracture that is not being well-visualized.

These fractures are in a different and generally less serious category than the other distal humerus fractures. Even with some displacement, there is usually a good result with closed treatment.

One of the most serious problems with the medial epicondyle fracture is that the avulsed bony fragment can be trapped in the joint. It is not common, but consider this when looking at plain films of a patient with a rigidly held, severely painful elbow with no clear fracture line. The medial epicondylar piece can be quite small and may be obscured on one view. If this seems to be the case, the fragment must be removed. This may be accomplished closed. Call the orthopedist for this.

Medial epicondylar fractures, displaced up to 1 cm, can be put into a long-arm splint (see Fig. 14-11) and the patient sent home after you call the orthopedist. Follow-up should be within 2 days.

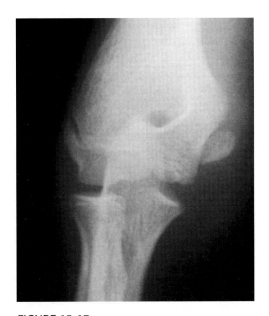

FIGURE 15-13

Medial epicondylar fracture.

Humeral Shaft Fractures (Fig. 15-14)

These fractures that often are associated with a radial nerve injury. Check for wrist dorsiflexion power and radial skin sensation with all humerus shaft fractures.

Fractures above the supracondylar region and below the surgical neck of the humerus heal remarkably well with closed treatment. Simple immobilization in splints reliably produces excellent functional and cosmetic results despite shortening and angulation. In general, the shaft and upper humerus are as forgiving as the distal humerus is unforgiving.

Although surgery is rarely necessary, these patients often must be admitted to the hospital for nursing care. The humerus is a big bone, the fracture is quite painful, and patients are often old and fragile. They seem to be "undone" by this fracture to a much greater extent than expected.

Some fractures of the shaft do fare better with internal fixation. These are segmental—i.e., there are two fractures of the humerus, leaving a free segment floating in the middle. The other relative indications for performing acute surgical fixation of a shaft fracture include the "floating elbow," which is a humeral shaft fracture in the presence of a "both bones" fracture of the forearm and severe multiple trauma.

The radial nerve wraps around the distal third of the humerus. It is essentially in direct contact with the bone at a location where there is common spiral-pattern fracture. This is called a *Holstein-Lewis fracture* (see Fig. 15-14*B*), and the patient is likely to have a wrist drop and numbness on the dorsum of the hand. Emergency surgery is not usually indicated; the nerve injury often improves spontaneously. You should,

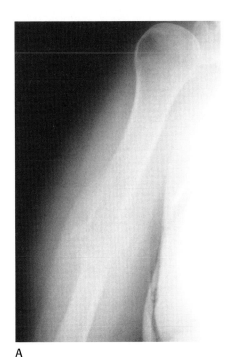

A

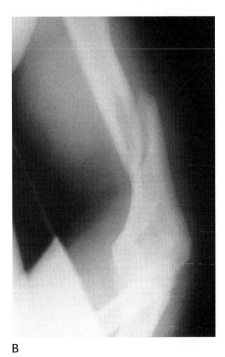

B

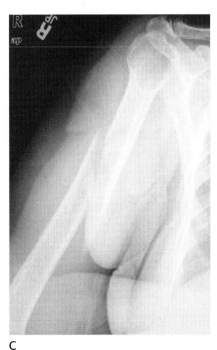

C

FIGURE 15-14

Humeral shaft fracture. *A.* Pathologic fracture. *B.* Holstein-Lewis pattern. *C.* Long oblique shaft fracture.

nevertheless, call the orthopedist immediately, document well, and be sure that the fracture is splinted.

Fractures of the shaft should be placed into a humeral sugar-tong splint. This is also called a *coaptation splint* (Fig. 15-15). Such splints are then supported by a sling, and patients are given instructions to sleep in an easy chair or sitting up in bed with pillows supporting everything. Try to mold in reduction as the plaster is hardening. This means that the AP and lateral films should be hanging up on the view box in front of you where you are working. Warn patients that the arm is going to turn purple as the bleeding from the fracture seeps to the surface. Also reassure them that the purple will disappear eventually. Notify the orthopedist on call.

Put the splinted arm into a sling. Pad the strap where it goes over the opposite shoulder. Feel free to wrap a 6-in. Ace bandage around the chest holding the

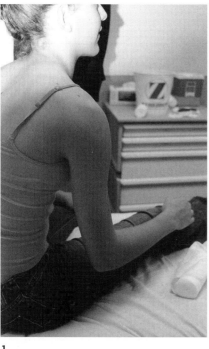

1

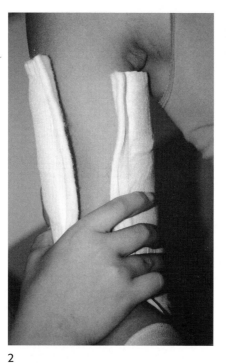

2

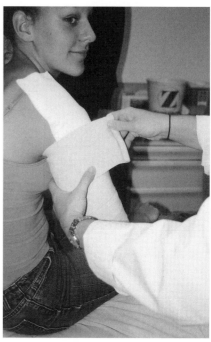

3

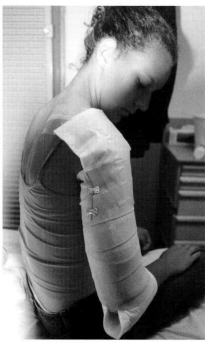

4

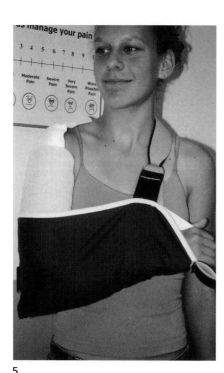

5

FIGURE 15-15

Coaptation splinting of the humeral shaft.

arm snug to the body if the patient is insecure. Just make sure that it does not limit motion of the chest in breathing. Also make sure that the patient is going to be able to take care of himself or herself at home with all this immobilization. Give instructions on hand and wrist motion—opening and closing the hand, curling and straightening the fingers, and extending the wrist all will help to prevent a stiff hand. Pain medication, ice, and 36-h follow-up with the orthopedist are needed before the patient can go home. Remember that sometimes all this is overwhelming to the patient, and despite insurance guidelines denying inpatient care, you will find it ethically impossible to send the patient home. Just make sure to keep the orthopedist, who must take the heat for this admission, aware of your findings.

CHAPTER

16

Shoulder and Proximal Humerus

NORMAL RADIOGRAPHS

Figure 16-1 shows the shoulder with labels for shaft of the humerus, surgical neck, greater and lesser tuberosities, humeral head, articular surface, anatomic neck, coracoid, acromion, and glenoid. Figure 16-2 is an axillary view of a normal shoulder showing the biceps groove (intertubercular sulcus). Figure 16-3 shows how to shoot an axillary view. Figure 16-4 shows the surface anatomy.

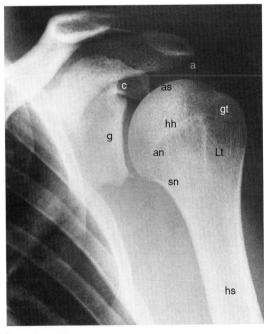

A

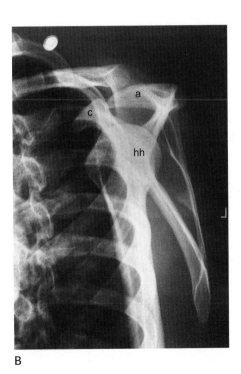

B

FIGURE 16-1

Normal shoulder. *A.* Anteroposterior (AP) view. *B.* Lateral view. hs = humeral shaft; sn = surgical neck; gt = greater tuberosity; lt = lesser tuberosity; hh = humeral head; as = articular surface; an = anatomic neck; c = coracoid process; a = acromion; g = glenoid.

FIGURE 16-2

Normal shoulder, axillary view. hs = humeral shaft; sn = surgical neck; gt = greater tuberosity; lt = lesser tuberosity; hh = humeral head; as = articular surface; an = anatomic neck; c = coracoid process; a = acromion; g = glenoid.

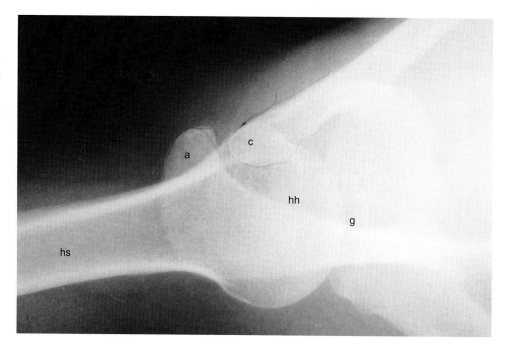

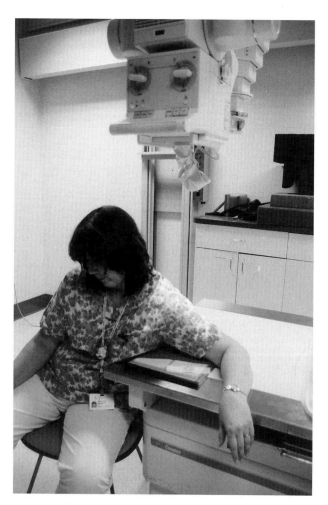

FIGURE 16-3

How to shoot an axillary view.

PROBLEM LIST

Fractures

- Fractures of the upper shaft
- Fractures of the surgical neck
- Fractures of the tuberosities, head, and neck

Dislocations

- Anterior dislocations
- Posterior dislocations
- Fracture-dislocations

Nonfracture Shoulder Pain and Dysfunction

- Acute subacromial bursitis
- Rotator cuff tears
- Calcific bursitis
- Acute acromioclavicular arthropathy

Upper Shaft Fractures (Fig. 16-5)

These are like midshaft fractures (described in Chap. 15), but they are harder to splint. It is difficult and uncomfortable to get the medial tong of the sugar-tong splint high enough into the axilla to actually control the fracture site. This turns out not to be a great problem because the outer tong and sling generally are sufficient. Like lower shaft fractures, these fractures can heal with a good deal of displacement and angulation

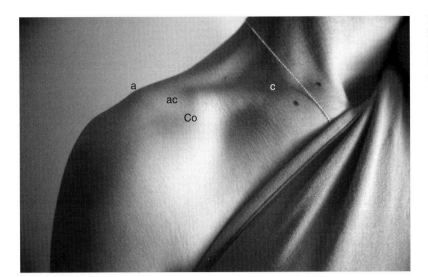

FIGURE 16-4

Shoulder surface anatomy. C = clavicle; ac = acromioclavicular joint; a = acromion; co = coracoid.

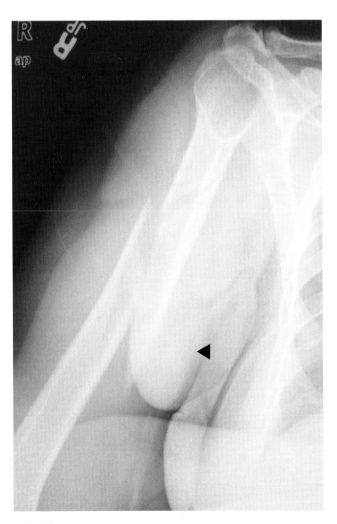

FIGURE 16-5

Proximal humeral shaft fracture. Arrowhead is at top of axilla.

with a perfect clinical result. Document the neurovascular status, apply splints and sling, and give pain medicine and instructions. You usually can send this patient home after notifying the orthopedist and arranging a 2-day follow-up. Do call the orthopedist, however, because some will recommend internal fixation.

Surgical Neck, Tuberosity, and Head Fractures

The surgical neck is something that only the humerus has. It is just distal to the tuberosities. This is the most frequently fractured part of the humerus—you probably will see as many surgical neck fractures as all the other humeral fractures put together.

Surgical neck fractures commonly have associated fractures of the tuberosities and humeral head.

Most orthopedists use Neer's classification of all proximal humeral fractures, which divides them based on the number of parts produced by the fracture lines. The parts have to be angulated or displaced to count in this system. A fracture line may delineate them, but until there is 1 cm of displacement or 45° of angulation of that part, it does not count toward the classification. As you might guess, a good bit of difference of opinion has been found among qualified observers as to what degree of angulation and displacement are present in a given film. Simply getting orthopedists who trained under the same shoulder specialist to agree on how many parts there are on a given film is not always easy.

In the emergency setting, you need to be able to tell what parts are actually fractured—the orthopedist you

FIGURE 16-6

Surgical neck fracture of the humerus.

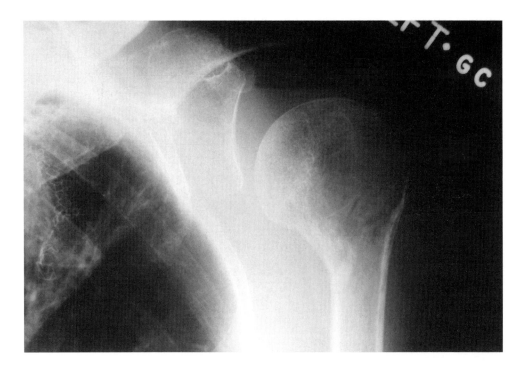

call needs to know about all the fracture lines, not just the displaced ones. There is value in describing, for instance, a "nondisplaced three-part fracture," although according to Neer's criteria, this is actually a one-part fracture.

The parts can be appreciated in the following radiographs.

1. The upper shaft of the humerus (Fig. 16-6)
2. The greater tuberosity (Fig. 16-7). This is the attachment of rotator cuff. This can be associated with typical anterior dislocation. In this film there is also a surgical neck fracture.
3. The lesser tuberosity (Fig. 16-8). This is the attachment of the subscapularis. This can be associated with the rare posterior dislocation.
4. The humeral head itself (Fig. 16-9). The articular surface is easily devascularized. Deformity produces glenohumeral arthritis.

Surgical treatment is indicated for most displaced fractures—either open reduction with internal fixation (ORIF) or, if the humeral head fragment has lost its blood supply, prosthetic replacement of the head with fixation of the tuberosities. It is possible to schedule this surgery within the next week, so some of these patients can be sent home in a sling with next day follow-up. Patients often are admitted for medical workup and surgery, though, so call the orthopedist to see if he or she wants to admit.

Nondisplaced fractures are treated with sling immobilization. A 6-in. Ace bandage swathing the arm to the chest is often appreciated for the first few days. Give pain medicine and instructions to sleep sitting up

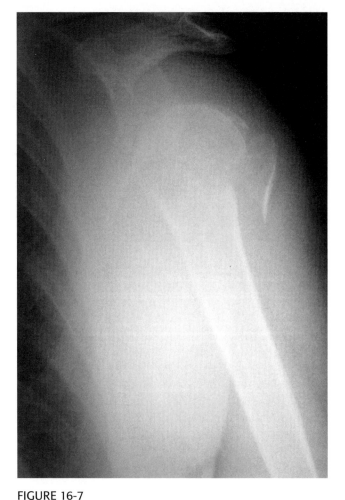

FIGURE 16-7

Greater tuberosity fracture.

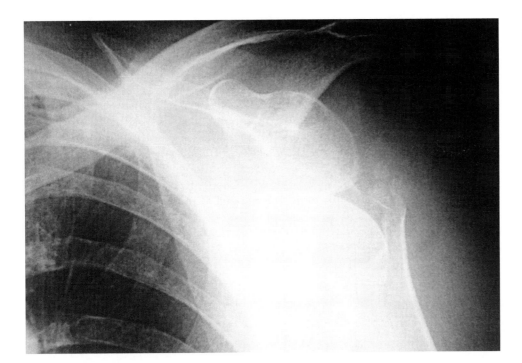

FIGURE 16-8

Four-part fracture showing the lesser tuberosity.

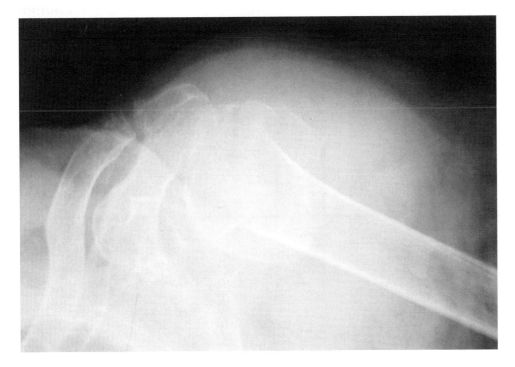

FIGURE 16-9

Fracture of the humeral head.

and to keep the hand and wrist from getting stiff. Many patients with nondisplaced shoulder fractures want to be admitted, and some really are unable to perform their activities of daily living with sling immobilization. You must make calls to the orthopedist, internist, and even social services personnel regarding such patients. Most insurance plans do not pay for inpatient admission for nonoperative shoulder fractures, so hospitals lose money admitting them.

Dislocations (Figs. 16-10 and 16-11)

Most dislocated shoulders present with anterior and inferior dislocation of the humeral head. You must get a plain film of the shoulder that you suspect is dislocated, no matter how many dislocated shoulders you have treated and no matter how confident the patient is of the diagnosis ("I've had this a million times"). Do note how the posterior aspect of the joint is less full and how when you put your fingers on the posterior angle of the acromion, the lack of humeral head is appreciable. Also be sure to note the neurologic condition of the upper extremity and ask the patient if the arm "went dead" or tingles. Elicit a complete history of shoulder problems, as well as the trauma that brought the patient in today. There are quite a few older people who live with a chronically dislocated shoulder, which you should not try to reduce in the emergency room.

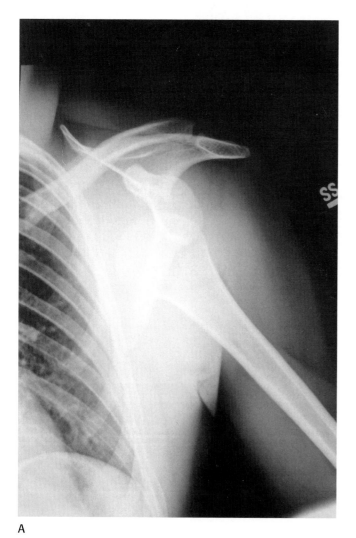

A

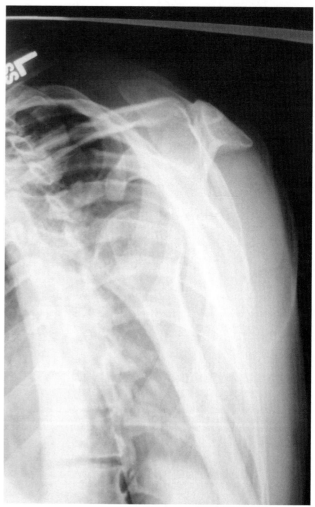

B

FIGURE 16-10

Anterior dislocation of the shoulder. *A.* AP view. *B.* Scapular lateral or "Y" view.

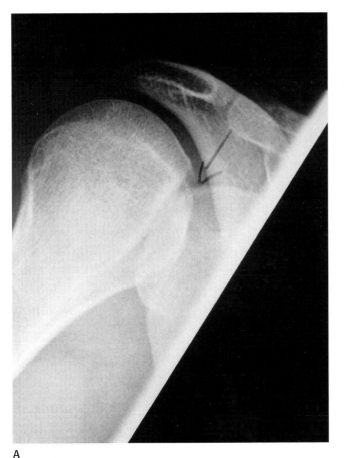

A

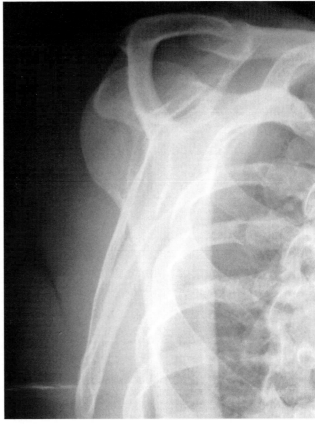

B

FIGURE 16-11

A. An AP view of the shoulder with posterior dislocation. Overlapping of humeral head and glenoid is suggestive but not diagnostic. *B.* Scapular "Y" view or scapular lateral view of same shoulder with posterior dislocation. The humeral head is clearly posterior to the glenoid.

As an emergency physician, you eventually will be quite comfortable reducing dislocated shoulders; they are common. You may very well become more adept at treating them than the orthopedist on call simply because you will do more emergency reductions.

Treatment: Dislocation

Most patients relax better with intravenous (IV) diazepam and morphine. Strong sedation generally is recommended (and used), but bear in mind that with sufficient cooperation it is possible to get many shoulders back in place without drugs. An injection of 10 ml of 1% plain lidocaine into the shoulder joint (Fig. 16-12) using a 22-gauge needle from posteriorly, below the posterior angle of the acromion, and making sure that it is deep to the cuff and deltoid before injecting is a fairly

safe and effective way of reducing the pain. Try this, along with a lot of reassurance, if you have concerns about using IV sedation.

The traction-countertraction method (Fig. 16-13) of reduction is used most frequently. It is not the easiest method but with sufficient help is safe and reliable. The Milch method (Fig. 16-14) requires either a cooperative or an unconscious patient. It does risk a fracture of the humeral shaft, but it is the easiest when it works. If you use it, be sure the patient is helping you with every move, and maintain a good bit of longitudinal traction as you *both* elevate the arm. The Stimson method (Fig. 16-15) puts the patient prone. It is uncomfortable and risky to leave a patient on his or her face with no side rails up. The Hippocratic method (Fig. 16-16) is safe and effective, especially if there is no one strong around to help

FIGURE 16-12

Injection of anesthetic into a dislocated shoulder.

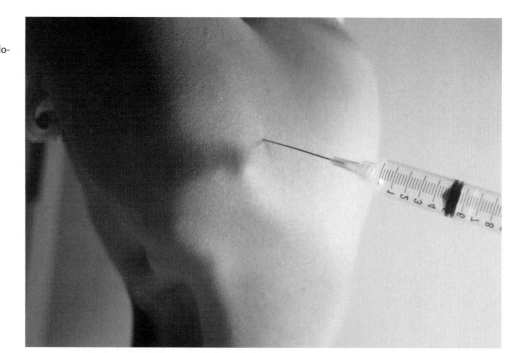

FIGURE 16-13

Reduction of a dislocated shoulder, traction-countertraction method.

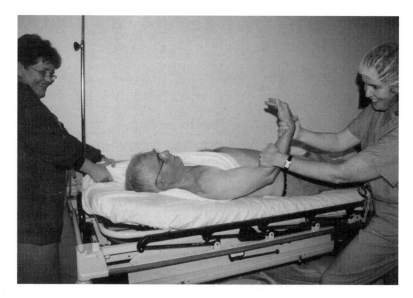

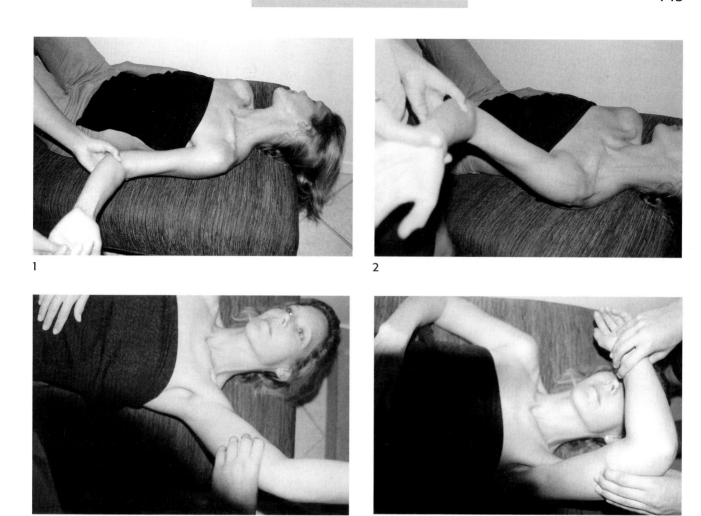

1

2

3

4

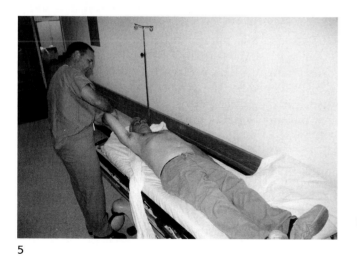

5

FIGURE 16-14

Reduction of a dislocated shoulder, Milch method.

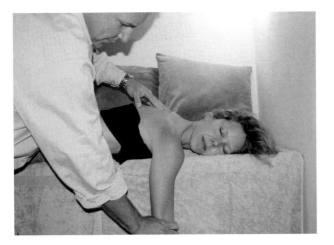

FIGURE 16-15

Reduction of a dislocated shoulder, Stimson method.

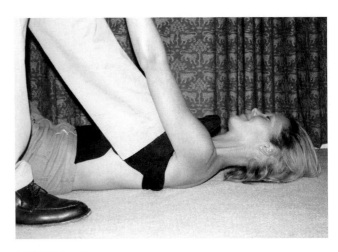

FIGURE 16-16

Reduction of a dislocated shoulder, Hippocratic method.

you. You must, however, establish a good, trusting relationship with the patient before climbing up on the stretcher and putting your smelly foot into his or her aching axilla.

When to give up and ask the orthopedist to come in to try to reduce this shoulder is a matter of personal judgment. The fact to keep in mind here is that the muscles fighting you eventually do fatigue, so it is common to get the reduction after trying hard and getting nowhere for half an hour or more. Your chances of success do not go down with the length of time you have been trying—they go up. This is a big part of the reason why, when you finally give up and call the orthopedist in, he or she seems to have such an easy time of it.

There is no shame in taking an acutely dislocated shoulder to the operating room for a closed reduction under general anesthesia if it cannot be reduced in the emergency room. Most patients welcome the idea after having suffered through all the pulling. This must be an orthopedist's decision, however, so let him or her be the first one to discuss it with the patient.

There is usually a satisfying "clunk" of reduction when the humeral head goes back into the glenoid, but not always. The patient is usually the one to tell you "it's back." A clunk also can be felt as the head rides up the glenoid but then falls back into the dislocated position—so don't trust noises. With the humeral head back, the posterior shoulder will feel full—like the other side—and rotation will not be so painful. Note these clinical signs of reduction, but always get a postreduction film, no matter how sure you are that it is back.

After reduction, the patient can go home with a sling, ice, pain medication, and instructions for a 3-day orthopedic follow-up. The sling is to be used at all times, including in bed. Showers can be taken with the arm held in the sling position. Sleeping sitting up is often more comfortable for the first few nights.

Older people (over age 50) with dislocations often have a torn rotator cuff. Younger patients usually have an intact cuff; the humeral head rips the anterior capsule of the shoulder off the anterior neck of the glenoid as it dislocates. This tearing away of the anterior capsule from its insertion on the glenoid is called a *Bankart lesion* (Fig. 16-17). You occasionally will see a small fracture of the anterior glenoid, a chunk of bone avulsed with the anterior capsule. This *bony Bankart* is something to tell the orthopedist about, but your treatment is the same. The divot or impression fracture that is left in the posterosuperior part of the humeral head by the inferior rim of the glenoid while the head is dislocated and wedged under the glenoid is called a *Hill-Sachs lesion*. When you see this divot on a plain film, you know for sure that the shoulder has been dislocated (Fig. 16-18).

Unusual Dislocations: Posterior and Inferior

The two unusual dislocations that should be kept in mind are the posterior dislocation and luxatio erecta. Posterior dislocations are associated with seizures, electrical shock, direct trauma to the shoulder, and having had a shoulder replacement. Their hallmark is inability to externally rotate the arm. The AP film is

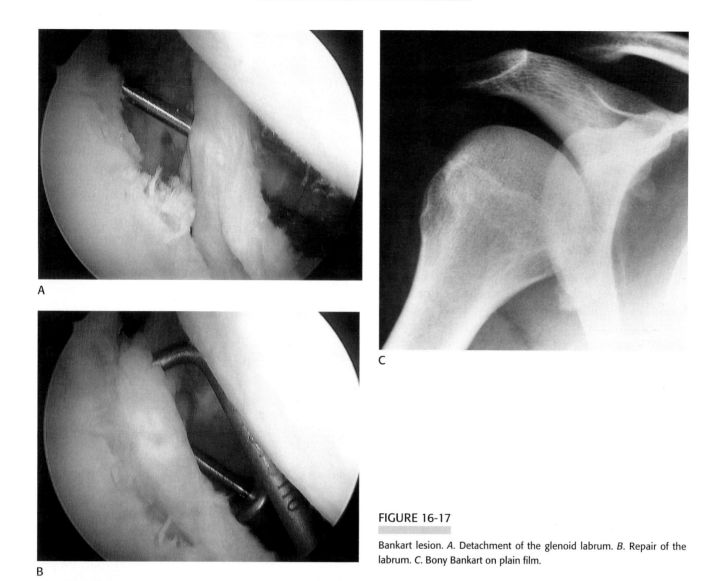

A

B

C

FIGURE 16-17

Bankart lesion. *A.* Detachment of the glenoid labrum. *B.* Repair of the labrum. *C.* Bony Bankart on plain film.

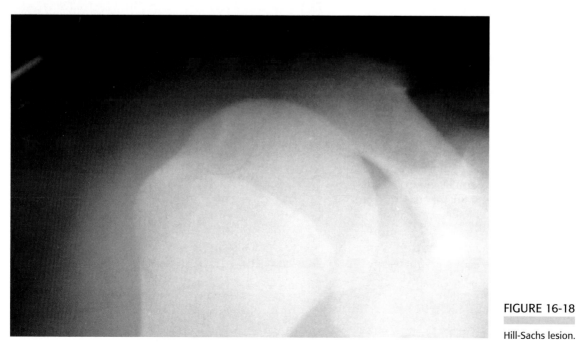

FIGURE 16-18

Hill-Sachs lesion.

suggestive but not diagnostic. You must get a scapular lateral or axillary view to see that the humeral head is posterior to the glenoid (see Fig. 16-11A, B). Luxatio erecta is easy to diagnose; the patient presents with the arm overhead. Plain films (a simple AP) will show clearly an empty glenoid with the humeral head displaced inferiorly.

These unusual dislocations are sufficiently rare and the orthopedist on call probably will want to see them. Call him or her as soon as you make these diagnoses. If the posterior dislocation is acute, it is relatively easy to reduce with traction. Take a careful history. A good number of posterior dislocations are chronic, and you will not be able to reduce these in the emergency room.

Luxatio erecta is often associated with severe neurovascular injury; the patient is writhing in pain and wants something done immediately. Traction in line with the arm as it lies is generally effective in reducing the pain. Help with countertraction (using sheets or just hanging on) and sedation are needed.

Fracture-Dislocations

A dislocation with any fracture of the upper humerus is called a *fracture-dislocation*. The most common is anterior dislocation with a fracture of the greater tuberosity (Fig. 16-19). Remember that this is the insertion site of the rotator cuff—this injury is therefore a dislocation in association with a cuff tear through bone. Treat this like any other anterior dislocation. Reduce it the same way. You probably will find that the tuberosity is reduced or nearly reduced when you check the postreduction films. Send the patient home with a sling, ice, pain medication, and instructions for a 2-day orthopedic follow-up.

Most other fracture-dislocations end up needing surgery because they involve displaced fractures of the humeral head and neck (Fig. 16-20). When the humeral neck or head is fractured, you will not be able to control them well by pulling on the patient's arm—the humeral shaft is not connected to the dislocated head. The reduction has to be accomplished surgically. These patients generally are admitted. Your treatment in the emergency room should include a sling and pillow to support the arm, neurovascular checks, sitting position, ice, and plenty of pain medication.

An anterior dislocation with a Hill-Sachs humeral head impression fracture, though in a sense a fracture-dislocation, is simply treated as an anterior dislocation.

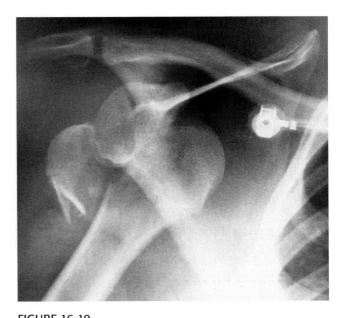

FIGURE 16-19

Anterior dislocation with a fracture of the greater tuberosity.

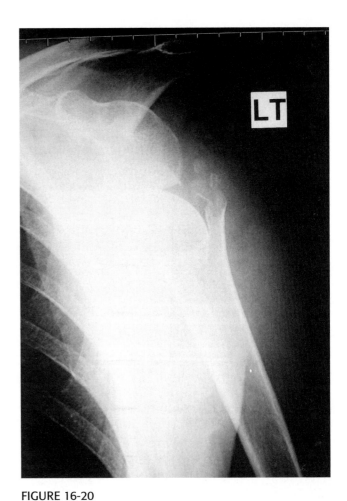

FIGURE 16-20

Four-part fracture-dislocation.

Acute Shoulder Pain without Fracture or Dislocation

Shoulder pain in a patient with neither fracture nor dislocation is a common presentation in the emergency department. Here is a list of the most common causes, in rough order of their frequency, with diagnostic clues. Do not forget visceral pains that refer to the shoulder, i.e., angina, aneurysms, and subdiaphragmatic irritation.

- *Cervical radiculopathy.* This is pain in the trapezius area, around the shoulder, and importantly, in the neck. There are paresthesias to the arm and hand. Pain increases with certain movements of the neck. The shoulder is nontender.
- *Rotator cuff pain.* This pain is worse at night and with overhead use of arm. The impingement maneuver is painful (Fig. 16-21). The anterior subacromial area is tender, and you may see calcium deposits in the subacromial space on plain film. Elevation of the arm is weak and/or painful with pain felt in the upper arm, passive motion less than active motion.
- *Subacromial bursitis.* This is like cuff pain but very tender at edges of acromion (Fig. 16-22A). The patient is in acute pain and permits little, if any, motion at the shoulder. Calcifications may be present in the subacromial space on plain film if calcific bursitis is present (Fig. 16-22B), but remember, not all cases of acute bursitis are calcific, and the calcium you see may be old. The shoulder is hot and may be swollen. The patient does not permit movement.
- *Acromioclavicular (AC) arthritis.* There is tenderness at the AC joint. There is pain in this area with forced adduction of arm (bring elbow under chin).
- *Biceps tendonitis.* The long head is tender in the biceps groove. Pain is anterior.
- *Rupture of the biceps tendon.* Sudden pain is seen in the shoulder and arm with a big lump on the anterior arm.
- *Adhesive capsulitis.* This is a frozen shoulder. External rotation and abduction usually are lost first. There is a sense of "blocked" motion at ends of range of motion. It has an insidious onset—one day the patient realizes that "I just can't move my arm." It is worse in diabetics.
- *Arthritic flare.* Usually rheumatoid (patient usually will have history of rheumatoid arthritis). There is sometimes osteoarthritis with a pseudogout flare of calcium pyrophosphate crystalline deposition. The posterior joint, the inferior to posterior angle of acromion, is tender.
- *Septic shoulder.* The joint is full, swollen, hot, and tender. The patient is sick. There is a history of injection into the joint, immunocompromise, or sexually transmitted disease. Lyme disease is a consideration.

Of all these, only septic shoulder requires true emergency treatment. Blood cultures, admission blood work, and aspiration of the joint for culture and microscopic analysis of fluid are needed if you think the shoulder is infected.

Anti-inflammatories, sling immobilization, and orthopedic follow-up are needed for all the others. Ice, sleeping sitting up, and rest also help. Many patients will request a corticosteroid injection, and indeed, this is an effective treatment for acute inflammatory conditions, most of which these are. See Fig. 16-23 for how to perform a subacromial injection. Remember that a plain lidocaine injection (7 ml of 1% plain lidocaine

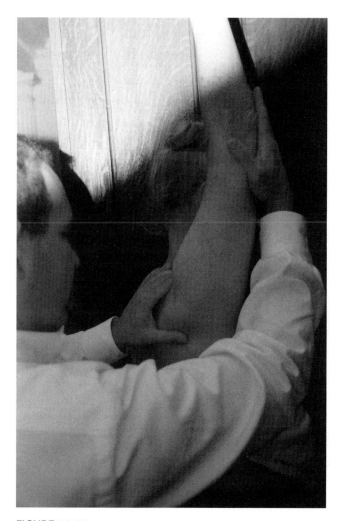

FIGURE 16-21

The impingement maneuver.

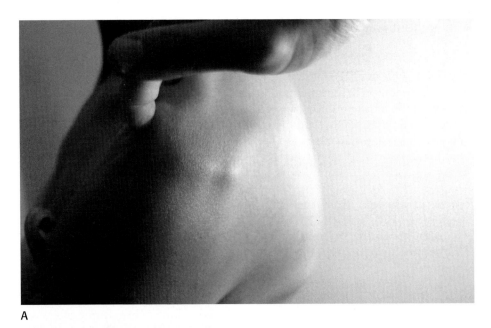

A

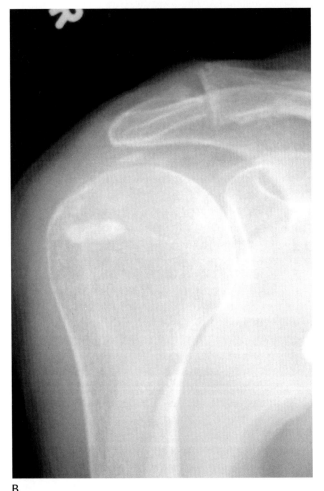

B

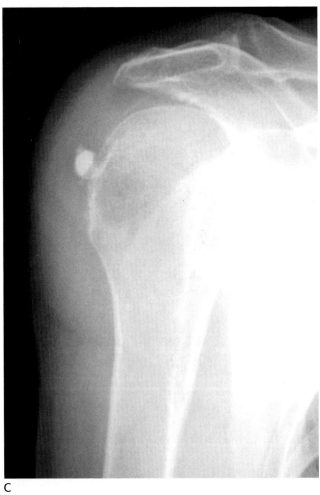

C

FIGURE 16-22

A. Anterior subacromial tenderness with subacromial bursitis. *B.* Calcification deposits in subacromial space. *C.* Calcification rotator cuff tendinopathy.

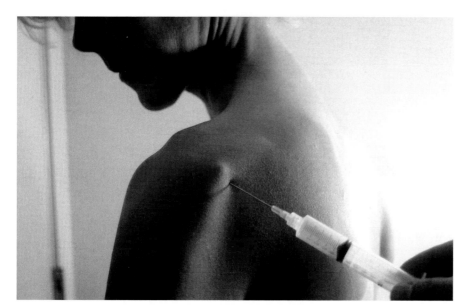

FIGURE 16-23

Subacromial injection technique.

into the subacromial space) can help quite a bit and does not risk cuff atrophy or susceptibility to infection as a corticosteroid might. Your decision, as an emergency physician, to get involved with steroid injections into shoulders you are not going to see again, hinges on a number of medicolegal, financial, and ethical factors. Most practitioners decide against doing steroid injections in the emergency room.

17

Clavicle and Scapula: Glenoid, Coracoid, Acromion, and Scapular Body

NORMAL RADIOGRAPHS

Figure 17-1 presents radiographs of a normal shoulder with labels showing the acromioclavicular (AC) joint, coracoid process, glenoid, acromion, shaft of the clavicle, body of the scapula, scapular spine, inferior angle. Figure 17-2 shows the anatomy. The clavicle is subcutaneous and S-shaped. The figure shows protraction, retraction, elevation, depression, rotation of the scapula, and the suprascapular notch.

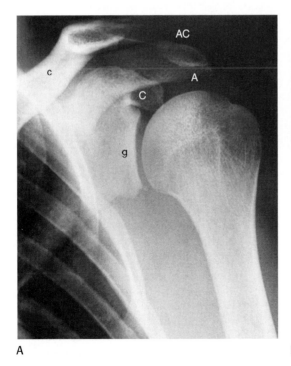
A

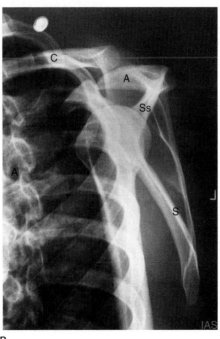
B

FIGURE 17-1

Normal shoulder and clavicle. AC = Acromioclavicular joint; CP = coracoid process; g = glenoid; A = acromion; C = clavicle shaft; S = scapular body; Ss = scapuler spine; IAS = inferior angle of scapula.

FIGURE 17-2

Surface anatomy of the scapula, shoulder, and clavicle. ac = Acromioclavicular joint; pa = posterior angle of acromion; C = clavicle; Sc = sternoclavicular joint.

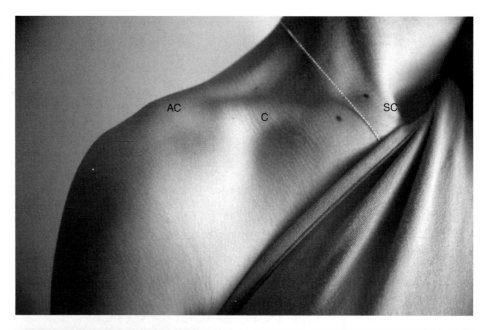

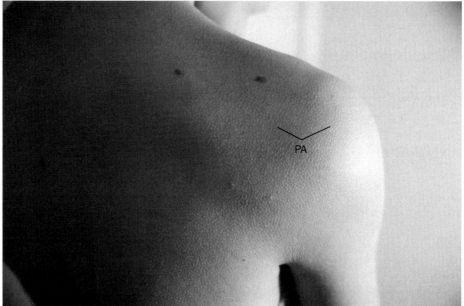

PROBLEM LIST

- Clavicle fractures
- Acromioclavicular (AC) separations
- Glenoid, coracoid, acromial, and scapular body fractures
- Sternoclavicular dislocation, subluxation

Clavicle Fractures

The clavicle is one of the most commonly fractured bones of the body. Clavicle fractures are difficult to re-duce and hold reduced. This is generally not a problem because they heal reliably, and a great deal of malre-duction is very well tolerated—usually leaving the pa-tient with only one problem, a bony lump where the fracture was, and this is generally less objectionable than the scar left by any attempt to reduce and hold the fracture surgically.

As long as the fracture is closed and there is no at-tendant injury to nerves, blood vessels, or the lung, pa-tients are well treated in the emergency room by putting the arm in a sling and applying a figure-of-eight Ace bandage or a McCloud-type clavicular brace (Fig. 17-3). The patient can be sent home with pain medication,

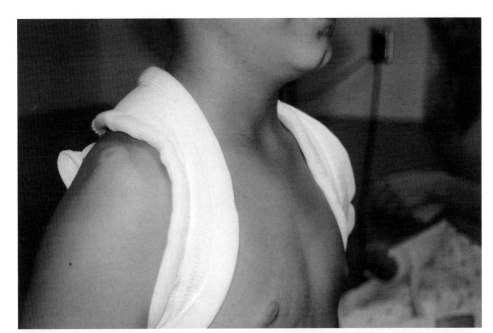

FIGURE 17-3

McCloud brace.

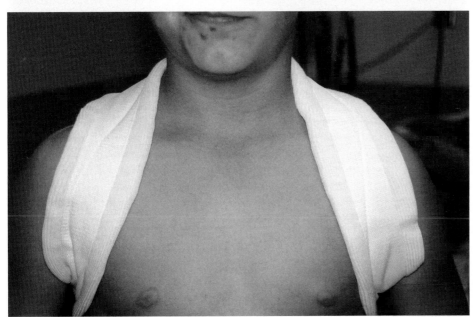

ice, instructions to sleep on the back with a small rolled towel between the scapulae, and orthopedic follow-up within 2 days.

A small percentage of distal clavicle fractures do require surgical reduction. These are fractures of the distal (outer) third that leave the coracoclavicular ligaments attached to the outer fracture fragment only. They essentially constitute an AC separation through bone and often produce a painful nonunion along with a "low shoulder" deformity. Such injuries do not need emergency surgery, however, because they are quite repairable for a few weeks. Do alert the covering orthopedist when one of these presents, however, because admission for surgery is a viable option (Fig. 17-4).

FIGURE 17-4

A. Fracture of the distal clavicle with coracoclavicular ligament injury.
B. Fracture of the shaft of the clavicle.
C. Fracture of the distal clavicle.

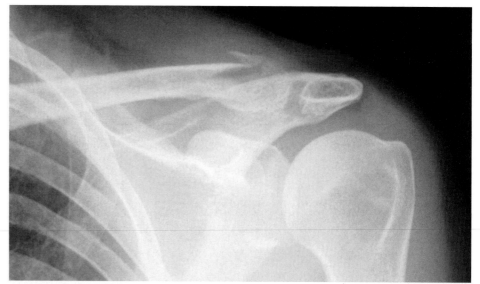

A

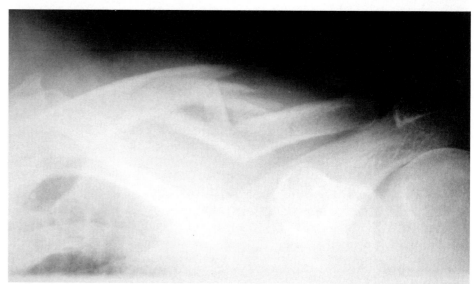

B

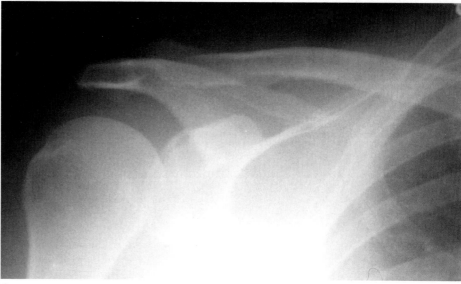

C

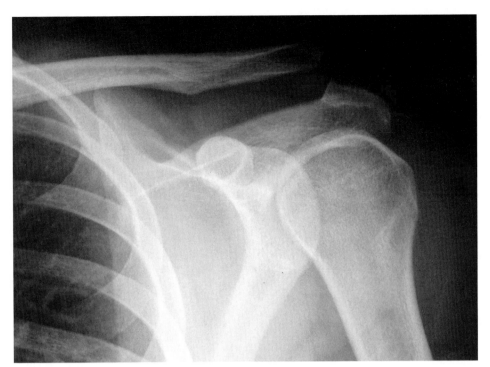

FIGURE 17-5

Acromioclavicular (AC) separation.

Acromioclavicular (AC) Separations (Fig. 17-5)

Generally, patients with AC separations have a history of a fall onto the shoulder with the arm at the side. The AC joint is tender and swollen. The most alarming aspect of this injury is that the injured shoulder may seem lower than the other one.

There is no fracture or dislocation on the anteroposterior (AP) shoulder film, only a variable degree of separation between the distal clavicle and the acromion. The degree of elevation of the clavicle relative to the acromion is the basis for grading these (grade 1: no elevation; grade 2: less than the width of the clavicle; grade 3: more than the width of the clavicle; and grade 4: grade 3 with posterior displacement). Bear in mind that the clavicle is not really elevated—it is the acromion that is depressed.

Put this patient into a sling, apply ice, check the neurovascular examination, and obtain plain AP radiographs of both shoulders. If the separation of the AC joint is not obvious, try measuring the distance from the coracoid to the clavicle. Compare this with the same distance on the other side. Look very carefully at the distal clavicle, searching for small fractures into the joint.

Although nearly all patients with AC separation injuries can be sent home from the emergency room with a sling, ice, pain medication, and instructions for a 2-day orthopedic follow-up. You should notify the covering orthopedist before the patient leaves. A growing consensus among shoulder surgeons suggests improved long-term results for AC separations treated surgically.

FIGURE 17-6

Glenoid fracture.

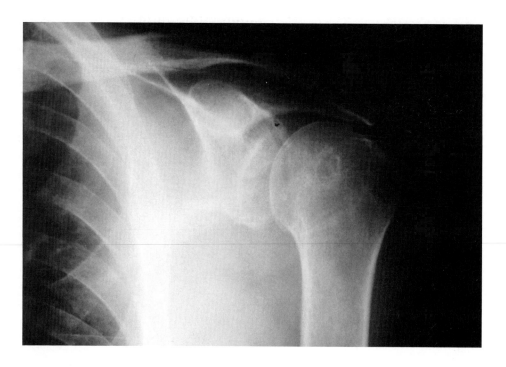

Fractures of the Glenoid (Fig. 17-6), Coracoid (Fig. 17-7), and Acromion and Scapular Body (Fig. 17-8)

These are all fairly unusual, but they are associated with direct local trauma to the shoulder area. They can be difficult to see on plain films. A computed tomographic (CT) scan of the shoulder frequently is obtained to better characterize these injuries.

The important issue with these fractures is their associated injuries. The patient with a scapular body fracture is likely to have broken ribs, a pneumothorax, or flail chest. An acromial fracture is produced by something hitting the top of the shoulder hard. Often stretch injuries of the brachial plexus and trapezius muscle are associated with acromial fractures. Coracoid base and glenoid neck fractures can injure the suprascapular nerve as it runs through its notch on the upper scapular body. This nerve gives motor power to the rotator cuff; thus the patient seems to have an acute cuff tear with paralysis or dysfunction of the cuff muscles.

If all these issues have been addressed, the treatment for these fractures in the emergency room is quite straightforward. Put the patient in a sling, provide ice and pain medication, and give instructions for 24-h orthopedic follow-up. Call the covering orthopedist to let him or her know about the patient. Few fractures of the scapula have been treated surgically in the past, but some are being operated on today for a variety of indications.

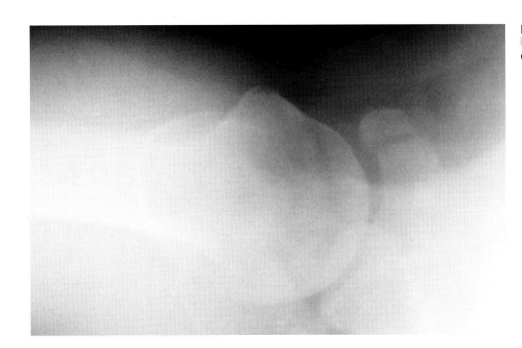

FIGURE 17-7

Coracoid fracture.

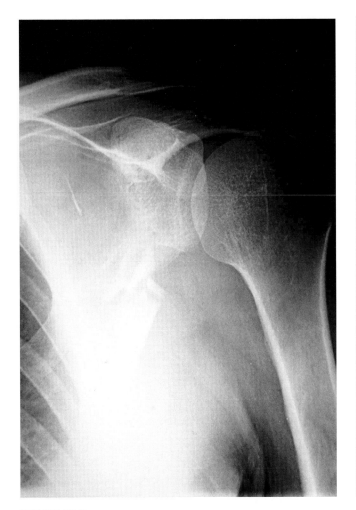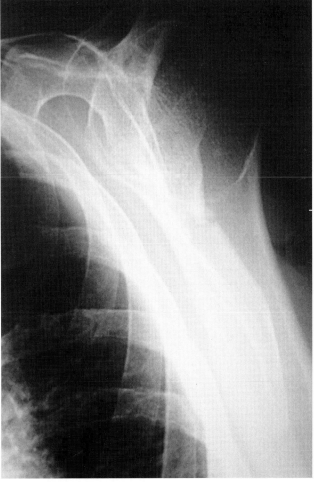

FIGURE 17-8

Scapular body fracture.

C H A P T E R

18

Open Fractures

Open or compound fractures are treated specially because of the risk of osteomyelitis. Bacterial infections of bone are very difficult to eradicate. Great care therefore must be taken with every compound fracture to minimize the risk of bone infection.

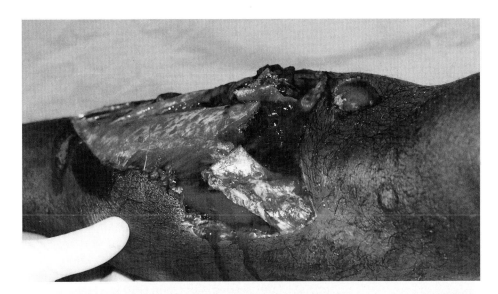

FIGURE 18-1

Grade III-B Open tibia-fibula fracture (knee is on right).

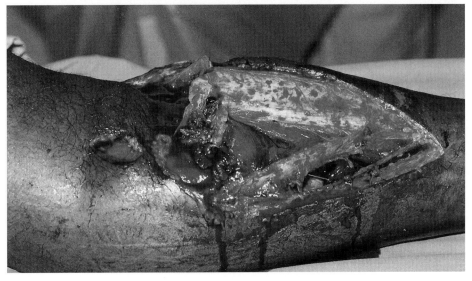

FIGURE 18-2

Grade III-B Open tibia-fibula fracture (knee is on left).

FIGURE 18-3

Grade III-B Open tibia-fibula fracture. Note dirt in medullary canal of tibia.

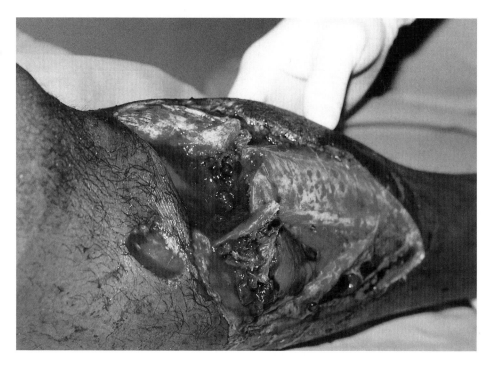

DIAGNOSIS

Even a pinhole through the full thickness of skin communicating with a fracture site makes a fracture *open*. Inspect every wound near a fracture very carefully. Wipe away any dirt, dried blood, or devitalized bits of skin. What appears to be only an abrasion often hides a small puncture wound. A laceration quite distant from the fracture site may still be a compounding wound because of the shifting and twisting of bone and skin that can take place during accidents. Most open fractures are obviously open fractures, see Fig 18-1, 2, and 3 but do be suspicious. When in doubt call it open.

CULTURES

The culture taken in the emergency room, before any antibiotics or antiseptics have been applied, has been shown to be the most valuable in predicting the responsible organism in case osteomyelitis eventually does develop. As soon as you recognize that a fracture is open, you should get a culture swab into the wound. If you need to probe a wound, consider doing it with a culture swab—getting both jobs done at once. If the patient has inadvertently been started on antibiotics before the culture is taken, tell the laboratory which antibiotic was used. There are antibiotic-removal culture media that can be used. You must be careful not to get any Betadine or other antiseptic into the culture; a tiny bit will keep anything from growing in the laboratory (but not, unfortunately, in the wound).

IMMOBILIZATION

This is important with any fracture but more so with compound ones. The less the bones move, the less contamination spreads. Splints, pillows, sand bags, and tape are needed immediately. Just make sure that you can still get to the wound.

ANTIBIOSIS

An intravenous (IV) antibiotic is begun as soon as cultures and immobilization are done. Remember that this is a prophylactic drug. A broad-spectrum antibiotic(s) is(are) needed. Cefazolin (1 g) is a legendary favorite of orthopedists. A patient with a penicillin allergy has a 95 percent chance of being totally fine with cefazolin, but pharmacies probably will balk if you order it. Cleocin (600 mg IV) is then the usual choice for penicillin-allergic patients. Anaerobic coverage is better with Cleocin, and if you have any reason to expect an anaerobic pathogen (human bite is one), Cleocin is a good choice. Fecal contamination or wounds on the sole of the foot (where *Pseudomonas* lives) need better gram-negative coverage. An aminoglycoside (e.g., gentamicin 60 mg) is the traditional choice.

CLEANSING

Cleansing an open fracture is tedious and requires discipline—it takes a long time. *All* visible contaminant, see Fig 18-3 must be removed, all nonviable tissue must be removed, and then 6 whole liters of irrigation, preferably under pressure, should be flushed through the wound, concentrating on taking every bacterium away from the bone. The emergency physician usually starts this procedure; the orthopedist finishes it in the operating room. Time counts with open fractures. When a particularly dirty one comes in, do not regard it as a museum piece to be kept in original condition to impress the orthopedist. Take a picture if you are that impressed, but start getting the dirt out of it immediately. This usually means doing the same things you would before suturing a dirty laceration: Remove gross dirt, sharply debride tissue margins, irrigate, and apply Betadine-soaked dressings. There is, of course, a limit to what should be done in the emergency room. The orthopedist must be called in stat as soon as the patient is admitted, and he or she must make the call on going to the operating room. Delays in getting to surgery will be much less likely to have disastrous consequences if as much cleansing as possible is done right away in the emergency room. Do not close any compounding wound or laceration with anything other than a single large tacking stitch to hold a flap in place.

OPEN FRACTURE CHECKLIST

- ABC's (airway, breathing, and circulation)
- Neuro/spine/visceral check
- Immobilize
- Culture and probe
- Apply Betadine dressing
- Start IV
- Give Kefzol/Cleocin/other antibiotic
- Send for x-ray
- Call orthopedist with diagnosis
- Begin cleansing

Index